FOOD VALUES

Sodium

OTHER BOOKS IN THE FOOD VALUES SERIES

FOOD VALUES

Sodium

Patty Bryan

PERENNIAL LIBRARY

Harper & Row, Publishers, New York

Grand Rapids, Philadelphia, St. Louis, San Francisco
London, Singapore, Sydney, Tokyo, Toronto

FIRST EDITION

Designed by Alma Orenstein

Library of Congress Cataloging-in-Publication Data

Bryan, Patty.
    Food values : sodium / Patty Bryan.
       p.   cm.
    ISBN 0-06-096444-8
    1. Food—Sodium content—Tables.   I. Title.
TX553.S65B79   1990
641.1′7—dc20   89-45634

90 91 92 93 94 AG/BC 10 9 8 7 6 5 4 3 2 1

Contents

Acknowledgments

I would like to thank Leah Wallach, who paved the way with the first three books in this series and provided much-needed advice and information for this one. I also want to thank the consumer affairs people at the many food manufacturers who provided information for brand-name products; Jean Stewart of the United States Department of Agriculture for her help with generic foods; Dr. Kelly Long of Rice University in Houston and Dr. William Henrich of the Southwestern Medical School in Dallas for their advice on the introductory material; Carol Hornig, nutritionist; and my husband for his help throughout. Kudos also to my agent, Joe Spieler, who helped with all the mail, and Carol Cohen and Eric Wirth at Harper & Row.

Introduction

Sodium occurs naturally in many foods, but the major source of the mineral in the American diet is common table salt, which is 40% sodium and 60% chlorine. In ancient times, wars were fought over a supply of salt because of its value as a preservative. A notable instance involving salt occurred when the British rulers placed a tax on salt in India in 1930. In response, Gandhi galvanized the populace and embarked on his famous march to the Indian Ocean to collect free salt. The episode was one of the first crises in the revolution that eventually brought down British rule in India.

In spite of the ancient allure of common salt, it was not until the early part of this century that its role as a *dietary* essential was established. And now that salt is almost universally available at a low price, and certainly so in the Western world, the main health problem associated with salt—sodium—has nothing to do with scarcity. We consume too much of it.

Why Do We Need Sodium?

Sodium is an essential mineral in the body. It is found predominantly in the vascular fluids within body vessels (arteries, veins, and capillaries) and in the fluids that surround cells. The remaining sodium is found within our bones.

Sodium is the major positively charged ion in the fluid outside cell membranes. It has many technical functions, but the main function of sodium affecting dietary habits is the role it plays in the regulation of total blood volume and therefore blood pressure. Sodium is readily absorbed into the bloodstream through the small intestine and the stomach. It is transported to the kidneys, filtered, and reabsorbed into the bloodstream if needed. Any excess sodium (and in the normal Western diet, at least 90% of the ingested amount is excess) is normally excreted in the urine.

Sodium and High Blood Pressure

The catch is that the excess sodium is not always excreted. We don't know exactly what happens but research indicates the following scenario as the most likely. The excess amount of sodium that the kidneys cannot handle is reabsorbed into the bloodstream. In order for the blood to maintain the proper concentration of sodium, more water must therefore be absorbed into the circulatory system. This greater volume of blood flowing through vessels that have not expanded increases the blood pressure. The result is the disease known as high blood pressure or hypertension.

Hypertension increases the risk of heart attack, stroke, and kidney disease. It is considered to be a primary risk factor in the development of cardiovascular disease, which, in all its forms, is the leading cause of death in the United States.

About one in four Americans has elevated blood pressure. Factors that increase the risk of hypertension include a family history of the disease, obesity—and high sodium intake. Because hypertension often produces no evident symptoms, blood pressure should be checked regularly. Some individuals can eat high-sodium diets without increased blood pressure; others cannot. We cannot predict who will develop the disease, but we know that almost all Americans eat much more sodium than their bodies actually require. Therefore, most health professionals believe that reducing sodium in the diet is sensible for the majority of Americans. For individuals with diagnosed hypertension, reduction of sodium intake is routinely prescribed, along with exercise, weight reduction if appropriate, and medication.

How Much Sodium Do You Need?

Sodium is essential, but you need very little. The dietary requirement for sodium varies from person to person and depends partially on the quantities lost in the urine, stools, and sweat. This amount is the minimum amount that must be replaced. It has been estimated to be about 15 milligrams per day. The National Research Council of the National Academy of Sciences suggests that a "safe and adequate" range of sodium intake per day is about 1,100 to 3,300 milligrams for adults. However, most Americans consume between 3,000 and 7,000 milligrams per day. The relationship between this fact and the high incidence of hypertension (one in four adult Americans) is not believed to be coincidental.

The opposite problem, sodium deficiency, causes a reduction of plasma volume, leading to an insufficient blood supply to vital organs. It can also cause a loss of body weight due to loss of sodium and water, muscle cramps, headache, and reduced milk production by lactating mothers. Symptoms may also include dizziness when standing, a consequence of low blood pressure.

However, this syndrome is uncommon because a diet too low in sodium is unusual. Nearly all foods contain some sodium, with meats containing especially high amounts. Elderly people eating "tea and toast" diets can sometimes consume a diet deficient in sodium. Also, certain strict vegetarian diets without salt present some danger of sodium deficiency.

Where Is Sodium Found in My Diet?

Sodium consumption falls into two main categories: naturally occurring sodium, known as "nondiscretionary" sodium, and sodium that is added during processing or preparation or at the table, which is considered "discretionary." It is important to note that the sodium in a TV dinner is considered "discretionary" even though the consumer at home has no way to remove it from the meal. The manufacturer had a choice in including the sodium in the product, and the consumer has the choice of buying something else.

Nondiscretionary Sodium Nondiscretionary sodium is present in varying amounts in many foods, but is more generally found in higher concentrations in foods in animal origin. Sodium content in a given food product is ranked low, moderate, or high. Foods that contain less than 100 milligrams of sodium per serving are low-sodium foods; foods with 100 to 250 milligrams per serving are considered moderate sources; any food with more than 250 milligrams per serving is considered a high-sodium source.

In general, fresh vegetables and fruits contain low to moderate amounts of sodium, while grain products, meats, and dairy products have moderate to high sodium content. But all of these amounts are lower than the discretionary sodium found in processed foods.

Discretionary Sodium The discretionary use of salt in commercial and home preparation and at the table varies greatly, but some experts believe that the American average of this discretionary sodium is about 2,000 milligrams, or as much as one half of the daily sodium intake.

Because a large and growing proportion of food is commercially prepared and processed, there has been an increase in the use of salt by industry and a decrease in home use. Salt, one of the original additives used by commercial food processors, is now second only to sugar in the amount used as an additive.

Salt helps prevent bacterial growth and spoilage in prepackaged foods. It provides special technical effects during food processing, such as ripening cheese and conditioning bread dough. But more commonly salt serves as a flavor enhancer.

Many other food additives also contain sodium. The following list of additives and their functions demonstrates how widespread the use of sodium is:

Baking powder—leavening agent

Baking soda—leavening agent

Monosodium glutamate—flavor enhancer

Sodium benzoate—preservative

Sodium caseinate—thickener and binder

Sodium citrate—buffer used to control acidity in soft drinks and fruit drinks

Sodium nitrate—curing agent in meat; provides color and prevents botulism

Sodium phosphate—emulsifier, stabilizer, and buffer

Sodium propionate—mold inhibitor

Sodium saccharin—artificial sweetener

Commercial foods that provide significant amounts of discretionary sodium in the diets of Americans include bread and bakery products, cured and processed meats, canned and frozen vegetables and milk products (especially many cheeses), sauces, soups, salad dressings, and many breakfast cereals.

The best way to show just how much sodium is added to processed foods is to compare a few before-and-after cases:

Raw potatoes have only 5 milligrams of sodium per 100 grams of weight, but the same weight of potato chips has 300 to 500 milligrams of sodium.

Cured ham has 20 times the amount of sodium in raw pork.

Fresh peas have less than 1 milligram of sodium per 100 grams, but frozen peas have 85 milligrams, and canned peas have 220 milligrams.

Watching sodium intake while eating at your favorite fast food restaurant can be a real challenge. Fast foods are often high in sodium and it isn't always easy to predict which foods provide the largest amounts. For example, an analysis of a typical McDonald's meal found that an order of regular salted french fries contained *less* sodium than the regular hamburger, the milkshake, or the fruit pie.

Watching your sodium intake and calorie consumption simultaneously is complicated because most reduced-calorie foods contain much more sodium than their nondietetic counterparts: salt, monosodium glutamate, and other sodium-rich items are used as flavor enhancers for these foods.

Most water supplies have less than 20 milligrams of sodium per liter, but in some areas of the country the sodium content of the water supply may be high enough—up to 220 milligrams—to make it an important source of the mineral, perhaps even to exceed the amount of sodium provided by food. Many of the ion-exchange units used in water softeners produce water with high sodium content. There is some evidence associating high sodium levels in water with incidence of atherosclerosis.

Sodium Labeling

Ingredient and nutrition labels can show you the major sources of sodium in your diet and help give you an idea of "the numbers." But for the individual concerned about sodium consumption or under doctor's orders to count the milligrams, there are unfortunate limitations in both labeling systems. It can be difficult, if not impossible, for the consumer to determine the precise sodium content in the diet.

The Ingredient Label   Ingredient labels are found on nearly all food products. They list the ingredients in relative order by weight, from the greatest to the least. The problem is that they provide no quantitative information. For example, the ingredient label for a processed ham on which the ham itself is listed above the salt tells us only that the ham weighs more than the salt! This is not a very helpful piece of information. Nor do these labels tell the consumer that ingredients such as soy sauce, mustard, catsup, and tartar sauce are high in sodium.

The Nutrition Label   The nutrition label is an advance, and many foods now have them. Placing sodium content on this label is optional unless the product claims to have a low- or reduced-sodium content, but many manufacturers are providing the optional sodium information as a service to consumers. The figure is given in milligrams (mg) per serving and includes the total figure for the product, combining discretionary and nondiscretionary sodium.

Avoiding Too Much Sodium

There are many ways to reduce sodium in your diet without sacrificing flavor or quality. Here are some suggestions. Remember that cutting back on sodium begins at the supermarket and continues through food preparation and serving.

At the Supermarket The surest, simplest rule is to buy fresh foods, which, as we have seen, are substantially lower in sodium levels. Most convenience foods have sodium compounds added, and many are quite high in total sodium content.

When choosing packaged foods, be a reader of labels. Learn to recognize all the sodium-containing ingredients, such as soy sauce. Know that, in general, less salt is added to frozen foods than to canned foods.

Many manufacturers are introducing foods with reduced sodium. Examples of types of foods that are now available in low-sodium form, or with reduced or no added salt, include canned vegetables, vegetable juices, sauces, canned soups, dried soup mixes, bouillon, condiments, snack foods (chips, nuts, pretzels), ready-to-eat cereals, bread and bakery products, butter, margarine, many types of cheeses, tuna, and some processed meats. These products can be more expensive. Make sure that reduction in sodium justifies the cost.

In the Kitchen Foods you prepare can and should contain less sodium than those that are commercially prepared. When you make foods from scratch, you can control how much sodium you add. A diet with less sodium does not have to be dull or limited in variety. Try new recipes that use less salt and fewer sodium-containing ingredients. However, substitutions cannot be made indiscriminately. Don't be fooled by recipes that have little or no salt but call for canned chicken broth, bouillon cubes, or condiments that do. Experiment with spices and herbs as seasoning instead of salt. Make your own condiments, dressings, and sauces. Adjust your favorite recipes for pastas, noodles, rice, and hot cereals by cutting down on the salt a little at a time. Your palate will accept this ploy.

These measures might take a little more time and effort in the kitchen, but the product will not only have decreased sodium; it will also probably taste better than the commercial brand.

And be sensible. The *total* amount of sodium in the diet is the number that counts. Eating a high-sodium food occasionally is not necessarily a problem.

At the Table   The seasoning of food is largely habit, so the first step in reducing discretionary sodium intake at the table might be simply to suggest that everyone at the table first *taste* the food before pouring on the salt. They might be surprised to learn that additional salt is unnecessary, especially on your new, improved recipes. A more drastic measure is removal of the saltshaker from the table. If this is politically impossible, substitute a salt mill, which takes more time to grind and delivers less salt.

How to Use This Book

Food Values: Sodium provides the number of milligrams of sodium and the total number of calories for thousands of foods.

The foods are divided into forty-eight categories covering all the things we eat and drink. As you flip through the pages of this book you'll quickly see where various foods are located. If you can't find a food in the category where you think it belongs, check the head note at the beginning of the category or refer to the table of contents. When products could be classified, we have tried to include a "see also" reference.

Each category begins with an alphabetical listing of generic food items, with fresh products listed before processed foods: for instance, you'll find fresh peaches before canned peaches. Following the generic foods are all brand-name products alphabetized by the name that is most easily recognized—either the name of the manufacturing company, of the product line, or of the product itself. For instance, Campbell's soups are listed under Campbell, the company names; Ortega sauces are listed under Ortega, the product line, rather than the manufacturer, Nabisco; and Kit Kat candy bar is listed under Kit Kat, because it is better known by its product name than by the fact that it is a Hershey product. Under each brand name, specific products are generally listed alphabetically: Aunt Jemima French toast, for example, precedes Aunt Jemima pancakes. We found, however, as most alphabetizers do, that some items could be listed in more than one way; we had to make choices. Fleischmann's diet margarine follows Fleischmann's regular margarine, for instance, and split peas are under *s*, not *p*. If you don't find a food under the first letter of the first word of its name, try looking for it under the first letter of another word in the name. The cross-reference should help here too.

Be sure to look for foods in the form in which you eat them: the way foods are prepared changes their nutrient values. Potato chips, baked potatoes, and potato soup all have different amounts of sodium.

We've used the portion sizes the Americans use—cups, ounces, or serving units—and when available, we've used two kinds of measures: for example, "3 cookies = 1 oz." Serving units are the easiest portions to measure; it's easier to count cookies than to weigh them. However, you can compare only serving units of the same weight. If a package of Brand X frozen lasagna weighs 10 ounces and a package of Brand Y frozen lasagna weighs 18 ounces, Brand Y will probably contain more calories and sodium per portion because it is larger. But Brand Y might contain fewer calories and less sodium per ounce. To compare two products of different sizes, divide the values for each product by the number of ounces they contain, and then compare the values for 1 ounce.

Also note the difference between weight measures and volume measures. Measuring cups measure fluid ounces. An ounce of water by weight fills a measuring cup to the 1-ounce line. But volume and weight are very different kinds of measure for solid foods. An ounce of unpopped popcorn, which is dense, wouldn't fill a measuring cup, for example, but an ounce of popped popcorn, which is airy, would fill more than one. In this book, portions for solid food given in ounces refer to weight. Fluid ounces (fl oz), cups (c), teaspoons (t), and tablespoons (T) refer to volume measurements. Since we don't ordinarily weigh our food, volume and weight measurements are given here when both are available and useful. For example, we've indicated how much of a measuring cup would be filled by an ounce of a given cold cereal when this information is available.

All values given here are approximations. No two apples, chicken breasts, or rolls are exactly alike. Data represent averages for several samples.

Figures provided by different sources may not be exactly comparable. The U.S. Department of Agriculture (USDA) and various manufacturers may use different procedures to analyze nutrient content and may round off the data in different ways. In the USDA *Composition of Food* series, our source of information about generic and fresh food, values are given to hundredths and thousandths. We rounded off figures for sodium and calories to the nearest whole unit. For example, we list 68.4 calories as 68 calories and 68.5 calories as 69 calories.

Many manufacturers use a simpler rounding-off system for calories, approved by the Food and Drug Administration, which regulates food labels. Calories between 0 and 20 may be given in increments of 2; between 20 and 50 in increments of 5; and above 50 in increments of 5 or 10. This means that there's no point in counting single calories when comparing products; a product listed as containing 197 calories, another as 195 calories, and a third as 200 calories may actually contain the same amount of food energy. For most practical purposes, these small differences don't matter. If you need about 2,000 calories a day, it doesn't matter if you get 2,005 one day and 1,991 the next.

This book contains the best and most complete information now available. Since food manufacturers constantly change recipes and product sizes and develop new products, some of the data contained here may quickly become outdated.

Calculating the Number of Milligrams of Sodium in Your Diet

To get an idea of how many milligrams of sodium are in your present diet, keep a record of everything you eat and drink for three days, preferably including one weekend day. Right after you finish a meal, snack, or cup of coffee, write down what you ate; how it was prepared; and the portion by volume (cups, tablespoons), weight (ounces, pounds), units (one medium apple, one English muffin), or all three if you can. To get a feeling for different food sizes, measure your food when you are at home. For example, instead of just pouring milk from the carton over your cereal, pour it into a measuring cup first to see how much you use. Use tablespoons to measure the milk you pour into your tea or coffee. You may find that the portion sizes used in the book are smaller than the ones you use. For example, for many American adults, a typical main course portion of spaghetti is 2 cups, not the 1 cup portion listed as a portion here.

At the end of three days, look up the sodium and calorie values for every food on your list. Add them up and divide by three to get your average daily intake.

The following salt-to-sodium conversions should help your calculations:

¼ t salt = 500 mg sodium

½ t salt = 1,000 mg sodium

1 t salt = 2,000 mg sodium

That last figure is the one to remember. One teaspoon from all sources is perfectly sufficient for a daily total.

Sources

1. *Food Values of Portions Commonly Used, 14th Edition*, Jean A. T. Pennington and Helen Nichols Church, Harper & Row, 1985.
2. *Nutritive Value of Foods*, U.S. Department of Agriculture, Nutrition Information Service, Home and Garden Bulletin #72, revised 1981.
3. *Composition of Food Series*, U.S. Department of Agriculture, Science and Education Administration:

   8-1 *Dairy and Egg Products*, revised November 1976.

   8-3 *Baby Foods*, revised December 1978.

   8-4 *Fats and Oils*, revised June 1979.

   8-5 *Poultry Products*, revised August 1979.

   8-6 *Soups, Sauces, and Gravies*, revised February 1980.

   8-7 *Sausages and Luncheon Meats*, revised September 1980.

   8-8 *Breakfast Cereals*, revised July 1982.

   8-9 *Fruits and Fruit Juices*, revised August 1982.

   8-10 *Pork Products*, revised August 1983.

   8-11 *Vegetables and Vegetable Products*, revised August 1984.

   8-12 *Nut and Seed Products*, revised September 1984.

   8-13 *Beef Products*, revised August 1986.

   8-14 *Beverages*, revised May 1986.

   8-15 *Finfish and Shellfish Products*, revised September 1987.

   8-16 *Legumes and Legume Products*, revised December 1986.

Information about brand-name products was supplied by the food processing companies themselves or taken from the above sources.

Abbreviations

c	=	cup
diam	=	diameter
g	=	grams
lb	=	pounds
mg	=	milligrams
oz	=	ounces
pkg	=	package
pkt	=	packet
T	=	tablespoon
t	=	teaspoon
tr	=	trace
w/	=	with
w/out	=	without
?	=	not available, or not known at this time
<	=	less than

FOOD VALUES
Sodium

	Portion	Sodium (mg)	Calories

❑ ALCOHOLIC BEVERAGES
See BEVERAGES

❑ BABY FOOD *See* INFANT & TODDLER FOODS

❑ BAKING INGREDIENTS

	Portion	Sodium (mg)	Calories
baking powder, sodium aluminum sulfate			
low-sodium	1 t	tr	5
straight phosphate	1 t	312	5
w/monocalcium phosphate monohydrate	1 t	329	5
w/monocalcium phosphate monohydrate, calcium sulfate	1 t	290	5
baking soda	1 t	821	0
candied fruit			
citron	1 oz	82	89
peel of grapefruit/lemon/orange	1 oz	5	89
cornmeal *See* FLOURS & CORNMEALS			
cornstarch *See* FLOURS & CORNMEALS			
flour *See* FLOURS & CORNMEALS			
pastry puff dough	1 oz	117	129
patty shell	2½ oz	210	240
piecrust			
from mix, w/vegetable shortening	for 2-crust 9″ pie	2,602	1,485
from sticks	⅙ double crust = 2 oz	400	290
frozen	¹⁄₁₆ crust = 1 oz	270	130
graham cracker	4.8 oz	184	159
homemade, w/vegetable shortening	for 9″ pie	1,100	900
yeast			
baker's, dry, active	1 pkg	4	20
brewer's, dry	1 T	10	25
torula	1 T	2	28

	Portion	Sodium (mg)	Calories

- **BRAND NAME**

Baker's
CHOCOLATE

	Portion	Sodium (mg)	Calories
German's sweet chocolate	1 oz	0	140
semisweet chocolate	1 oz	0	140
semisweet chocolate–flavored chips	¼ c	25	190
semisweet real chocolate chips	¼ c	0	200
unsweetened chocolate	1 oz	0	140

COCONUT

	Portion	Sodium (mg)	Calories
Angel Flake, bag	⅓ c	75	120
Davis			
baking powder	1 t	330	8
Hershey			
milk chocolate chips	1 oz	35	150
semisweet chocolate chips, regular & miniature	¼ c or 1½ oz	5	220
unsweetened baking chocolate	1 oz	5	190
Nabisco			
graham cracker crumbs	2 T	90	60
Reese's			
peanut butter–flavored chips	¼ c or 1½ oz	90	230
Sunshine			
graham cracker crumbs	1 c	990	550

❏ BAKING MIXES

cakes & pastries, prepared from mix *See* DESSERTS: CAKES, PASTRIES, & PIES
pancakes, prepared from mix *See* BREAKFAST FOODS, PREPARED
pie fillings, prepared from mix *See* DESSERTS: CUSTARDS, GELATINS, PUDDINGS, & PIE FILLINGS
waffles, prepared from mix *See* BREAKFAST FOODS, PREPARED

- **BRAND NAME**

Arrowhead Mills

	Portion	Sodium (mg)	Calories
biscuit mix	2 oz	170	100
bran muffin mix	2 muffins	330	270
corn bread mix	1 oz	220	100

	Portion	Sodium (mg)	Calories
Aunt Jemima			
Easy Mix coffee cake	1.3 oz	279	156
Easy Mix corn bread	1.7 oz	679	196
Dromedary			
corn bread, prepared	2″×2″ piece	480	130
corn muffin, prepared	1 muffin	270	120
gingerbread, prepared	2″×2″ piece	190	100
pound cake, prepared	½″ slice	160	150
Fearn			
BAKING MIXES			
brown rice	½ c	810	215
rice	½ c	960	260
whole-wheat	½ c	785	210
BREAD & MUFFIN MIXES			
bran muffin	1½ oz	375	110
corn bread	⅓ c dry	510	160
CAKE MIXES			
banana	⅓ c dry	450	130
carob	⅓ c dry	440	120
carrot	⅓ c dry	480	140
spice	⅓ c dry	495	140
Flako			
corn muffin mix	1 oz	351	116
pie crust mix	1.7 oz	393	241
Jell-O			
cheesecake, prepared w/whole milk	⅛ of 8″ cake	350	280
chocolate mousse pie, prepared w/whole milk	⅛ pie	440	250
coconut cream pie, prepared w/whole milk	⅛ pie	310	260
Pillsbury			
All Ready pie crust	⅛ of 2-crust pie	210	240
biscuits, bread, rolls *See* BREADS, ROLLS, BISCUITS, & MUFFINS			
Royal			
chocolate mint pie mix	⅛ pie	280	260
chocolate mousse pie mix	⅛ pie	260	230
lemon meringue pie mix	⅛ pie	250	310
lite cheese cake mix	⅛ pie	380	210
Real cheese cake mix	⅛ pie	370	280

	Portion	Sodium (mg)	Calories

❑ BEANS *See* LEGUMES & LEGUME PRODUCTS

❑ BEEF, FRESH & CURED
See also PROCESSED MEAT & POULTRY PRODUCTS

NOTE: "1 lb raw" refers to the edible portion of meat yielded when 1 pound of the raw product is cooked.

Beef, Fresh

BRISKET

Lean & Fat

	Portion	Sodium (mg)	Calories
whole, all grades, braised	3 oz cooked	52	332
	1 lb raw	198	1,258
flat half, all grades, braised	3 oz cooked	55	347
	1 lb raw	207	1,311
point half, all grades, braised	3 oz cooked	47	311
	1 lb raw	179	1,172

Lean Only

whole, all grades, braised	3 oz cooked	61	205
	1 lb raw	153	513
flat half, all grades, braised	3 oz cooked	66	223
	1 lb raw	161	549
point half, all grades, braised	3 oz cooked	54	181
	1 lb raw	137	461

CHUCK, ARM ROAST

Lean & Fat

all grades, braised	3 oz cooked	51	297
	1 lb raw	164	962
choice, braised	3 oz cooked	50	301
	1 lb raw	165	982
good, braised	3 oz cooked	51	287
	1 lb raw	159	894
prime, braised	3 oz cooked	50	332
	1 lb raw	162	1,082

Lean Only

all grades, braised	3 oz cooked	56	196
	1 lb raw	134	467
choice, braised	3 oz cooked	56	199
	1 lb raw	134	473
good, braised	3 oz cooked	56	189
	1 lb raw	131	439

	Portion	Sodium (mg)	Calories
prime, braised	3 oz cooked	56	222
	1 lb raw	126	499

CHUCK, BLADE ROAST
Lean & Fat

all grades, braised	3 oz cooked	53	325
	1 lb raw	158	961
choice, braised	3 oz cooked	53	330
	1 lb raw	159	982
good, braised	3 oz cooked	54	311
	1 lb raw	153	882
prime, braised	3 oz cooked	53	354
	1 lb raw	155	1,029

Lean Only

all grades, braised	3 oz cooked	60	230
	1 lb raw	129	492
choice, braised	3 oz cooked	60	234
	1 lb raw	130	503
good, braised	3 oz cooked	60	218
	1 lb raw	127	456
prime, braised	3 oz cooked	60	270
	1 lb raw	127	569

FLANK
Lean & Fat
choice

braised	3 oz cooked	61	218
	1 lb raw	191	689
broiled	3 oz cooked	70	216
	1 lb raw	278	863

Lean Only
choice

braised	3 oz cooked	61	208
	1 lb raw	188	635
broiled	3 oz cooked	70	207
	1 lb raw	274	808

GROUND BEEF
Extra Lean
baked

medium	3 oz cooked	42	213
	1 lb raw	170	863
well done	3 oz cooked	54	232
	1 lb raw	172	733

broiled

medium	3 oz cooked	59	217
	1 lb raw	234	859

	Portion	Sodium (mg)	Calories
broiled *(cont.)*			
well done	3 oz cooked	70	225
	1 lb raw	230	744
pan-fried			
medium	3 oz cooked	59	216
	1 lb raw	238	866
well done	3 oz cooked	69	224
	1 lb raw	238	777
Lean			
baked			
medium	3 oz cooked	47	227
	1 lb raw	187	899
well done	3 oz cooked	61	248
	1 lb raw	187	768
broiled			
medium	3 oz cooked	65	231
	1 lb raw	248	876
well done	3 oz cooked	76	238
	1 lb raw	250	785
pan-fried			
medium	3 oz cooked	65	234
	1 lb raw	251	901
well done	3 oz cooked	74	235
	1 lb raw	249	791
Regular			
baked			
medium	3 oz cooked	51	244
	1 lb raw	191	913
well done	3 oz cooked	63	269
	1 lb raw	189	804
broiled			
medium	3 oz cooked	70	246
	1 lb raw	251	880
well done	3 oz cooked	79	248
	1 lb raw	252	793
pan-fried			
medium	3 oz cooked	71	260
	1 lb raw	258	941
well done	3 oz cooked	79	243
	1 lb raw	257	792
GROUND, FROZEN PATTIES			
broiled, medium	3 oz cooked	66	240
	1 lb raw	242	882

	Portion	Sodium (mg)	Calories
RIB, WHOLE (RIBS 6–12)			
Lean & Fat			
all grades			
broiled	3 oz cooked	52	308
	1 lb raw	175	1,039
roasted	3 oz cooked	54	324
	1 lb raw	173	1,042
choice			
broiled	3 oz cooked	52	313
	1 lb raw	175	1,060
roasted	3 oz cooked	54	328
	1 lb raw	173	1,062
good			
broiled	3 oz cooked	52	289
	1 lb raw	174	969
roasted	3 oz cooked	54	300
	1 lb raw	174	978
prime			
broiled	3 oz cooked	51	347
	1 lb raw	177	1,199
roasted	3 oz cooked	53	361
	1 lb raw	175	1,189
Lean Only			
all grades			
broiled	3 oz cooked	59	194
	1 lb raw	140	461
roasted	3 oz cooked	63	204
	1 lb raw	138	449
choice			
broiled	3 oz cooked	59	198
	1 lb raw	139	469
roasted	3 oz cooked	63	209
	1 lb raw	137	456
good			
broiled	3 oz cooked	59	181
	1 lb raw	143	440
roasted	3 oz cooked	63	191
	1 lb raw	140	430
prime			
broiled	3 oz cooked	59	238
	1 lb raw	139	562
roasted	3 oz cooked	63	248
	1 lb raw	135	536

	Portion	Sodium (mg)	Calories
RIB, EYE, SMALL END (RIBS 10–12)			
Lean & Fat			
choice, broiled	3 oz cooked	55	250
	1 lb raw	211	966
Lean Only			
choice, broiled	3 oz cooked	58	191
	1 lb raw	190	623
RIB, LARGE END (RIBS 6–9)			
Lean & Fat			
all grades			
broiled	3 oz cooked	51	321
	1 lb raw	173	1,083
roasted	3 oz cooked	54	313
	1 lb raw	179	1,030
choice			
broiled	3 oz cooked	51	327
	1 lb raw	173	1,107
roasted	3 oz cooked	54	316
	1 lb raw	179	1,040
good			
broiled	3 oz cooked	52	301
	1 lb raw	174	1,009
roasted	3 oz cooked	54	304
	1 lb raw	179	1,000
prime			
broiled	3 oz cooked	51	361
	1 lb raw	178	1,267
roasted	3 oz cooked	54	346
	1 lb raw	176	1,136
Lean Only			
all grades			
broiled	3 oz cooked	59	198
	1 lb raw	135	453
roasted	3 oz cooked	62	207
	1 lb raw	146	487
choice			
broiled	3 oz cooked	59	203
	1 lb raw	135	464
roasted	3 oz cooked	62	210
	1 lb raw	146	495
good			
broiled	3 oz cooked	59	183
	1 lb raw	139	428
roasted	3 oz cooked	62	197
	1 lb raw	148	468

	Portion	Sodium (mg)	Calories
prime			
broiled	3 oz cooked	59	250
	1 lb raw	136	575
roasted	3 oz cooked	62	241
	1 lb raw	140	543

RIB, SMALL END (RIBS 10–12)
Lean & Fat

	Portion	Sodium (mg)	Calories
all grades			
broiled	3 oz cooked	53	277
	1 lb raw	181	950
roasted	3 oz cooked	56	305
	1 lb raw	179	981
choice			
broiled	3 oz cooked	53	282
	1 lb raw	181	965
roasted	3 oz cooked	55	312
	1 lb raw	178	1,002
good			
broiled	3 oz cooked	53	263
	1 lb raw	180	889
roasted	3 oz cooked	56	283
	1 lb raw	179	900
prime			
broiled	3 oz cooked	52	309
	1 lb raw	176	1,041
roasted	3 oz cooked	55	357
	1 lb raw	175	1,142

Lean Only

	Portion	Sodium (mg)	Calories
all grades			
broiled	3 oz cooked	58	188
	1 lb raw	153	492
roasted	3 oz cooked	64	201
	1 lb raw	148	465
choice			
broiled	3 oz cooked	58	191
	1 lb raw	152	499
roasted	3 oz cooked	64	206
	1 lb raw	147	476
good			
broiled	3 oz cooked	58	178
	1 lb raw	155	473
roasted	3 oz cooked	64	183
	1 lb raw	151	433
prime			
broiled	3 oz cooked	58	221
	1 lb raw	147	559
roasted	3 oz cooked	64	259
	1 lb raw	141	572

	Portion	Sodium (mg)	Calories
RIB, SHORT			
Lean & Fat			
choice, braised	3 oz cooked	43	400
	1 lb raw	114	1,064
Lean Only			
choice, braised	3 oz cooked	50	251
	1 lb raw	72	363
ROUND, FULL CUT			
Lean & Fat			
choice, broiled	3 oz cooked	51	233
	1 lb raw	183	832
good, broiled	3 oz cooked	51	222
	1 lb raw	182	790
Lean Only			
choice, broiled	3 oz cooked	54	165
	1 lb raw	162	493
good, broiled	3 oz cooked	54	157
	1 lb raw	163	470
ROUND, BOTTOM			
Lean & Fat			
all grades, braised	3 oz cooked	43	222
	1 lb raw	140	725
choice, braised	3 oz cooked	43	224
	1 lb raw	140	734
good, braised	3 oz cooked	43	215
	1 lb raw	140	700
prime, braised	3 oz cooked	43	253
	1 lb raw	144	853
Lean Only			
all grades, braised	3 oz cooked	44	189
	1 lb raw	131	564
choice, braised	3 oz cooked	44	191
	1 lb raw	131	571
good, braised	3 oz cooked	44	182
	1 lb raw	131	543
prime, braised	3 oz cooked	44	212
	1 lb raw	128	622
ROUND, EYE OF			
Lean & Fat			
all grades, roasted	3 oz cooked	50	206
	1 lb raw	212	869

	Portion	Sodium (mg)	Calories
choice, roasted	3 oz cooked	50	207
	1 lb raw	211	871
good, roasted	3 oz cooked	50	201
	1 lb raw	213	851
prime, roasted	3 oz cooked	51	213
	1 lb raw	211	888
Lean Only			
all grades, roasted	3 oz cooked	52	155
	1 lb raw	194	575
choice, roasted	3 oz cooked	52	156
	1 lb raw	194	578
good, roasted	3 oz cooked	52	151
	1 lb raw	195	562
prime, roasted	3 oz cooked	52	168
	1 lb raw	196	628
ROUND, TIP			
Lean & Fat			
all grades, roasted	3 oz cooked	53	213
	1 lb raw	203	823
choice, roasted	3 oz cooked	53	216
	1 lb raw	204	837
good, roasted	3 oz cooked	53	205
	1 lb raw	201	780
prime, roasted	3 oz cooked	52	242
	1 lb raw	201	932
Lean Only			
all grades, roasted	3 oz cooked	55	162
	1 lb raw	186	546
choice, roasted	3 oz cooked	55	164
	1 lb raw	186	552
good, roasted	3 oz cooked	55	156
	1 lb raw	186	524
prime, roasted	3 oz cooked	55	181
	1 lb raw	181	593
ROUND, TOP			
Lean & Fat			
all grades, broiled	3 oz cooked	51	179
	1 lb raw	199	701
choice			
broiled	3 oz cooked	51	181
	1 lb raw	200	709
pan-fried	3 oz cooked	57	246
	1 lb raw	188	819
good, broiled	3 oz cooked	51	176
	1 lb raw	199	686
prime, broiled	3 oz cooked	51	201
	1 lb raw	198	783

	Portion	Sodium (mg)	Calories
Lean Only			
all grades, broiled	3 oz cooked	52	162
	1 lb raw	194	610
choice			
broiled	3 oz cooked	52	165
	1 lb raw	194	617
pan-fried	3 oz cooked	60	193
	1 lb raw	173	556
good, broiled	3 oz cooked	52	156
	1 lb raw	192	583
prime, broiled	3 oz cooked	52	183
	1 lb raw	191	678
SHANK CROSSCUTS			
Lean & Fat			
choice, simmered	3 oz cooked	52	208
	1 lb raw	128	508
Lean Only			
choice, simmered	3 oz cooked	54	171
	1 lb raw	120	380
SHORT LOIN, PORTERHOUSE STEAK			
Lean & Fat			
choice, broiled	3 oz cooked	52	254
	1 lb raw	165	803
Lean Only			
choice, broiled	3 oz cooked	56	185
	1 lb raw	145	483
SHORT LOIN, T-BONE STEAK			
Lean & Fat			
choice, broiled	3 oz cooked	51	276
	1 lb raw	164	888
Lean Only			
choice, broiled	3 oz cooked	56	182
	1 lb raw	137	447
SHORT LOIN, TENDERLOIN			
Lean & Fat			
all grades			
broiled	3 oz cooked	52	226
	1 raw steak, edible portion = 4 oz	70	306

	Portion	Sodium (mg)	Calories
roasted	3 oz cooked	47	258
	1 raw steak, edible portion = 4.2 oz	67	364
choice			
broiled	3 oz cooked	51	230
	1 raw steak, edible portion = 4.1 oz	70	314
roasted	3 oz cooked	47	262
	1 raw steak, edible portion = 4.2 oz	67	370
good			
broiled	3 oz cooked	52	216
	1 raw steak, edible portion = 4 oz	69	286
roasted	3 oz cooked	48	245
	1 raw steak, edible portion = 4.2 oz	67	343
prime			
broiled	3 oz cooked	50	270
	1 raw steak, edible portion = 4 oz	67	362
roasted	3 oz cooked	47	305
	1 raw steak, edible portion = 4.1 oz	63	416
Lean Only			
all grades			
broiled	3 oz cooked	54	174
	1 raw steak, edible portion = 3½ oz	63	204
roasted	3 oz cooked	50	186
	1 raw steak, edible portion = 3½ oz	58	215
choice			
broiled	3 oz cooked	54	176
	1 raw steak, edible portion = 3.6 oz	64	209
roasted	3 oz cooked	50	189
	1 raw steak, edible portion = 3.4 oz	57	216

	Portion	Sodium (mg)	Calories
good			
broiled	3 oz cooked	54	167
	1 raw steak, edible portion = 3½ oz	63	196
roasted	3 oz cooked	50	177
	1 raw steak, edible portion = 3½ oz	59	206
prime			
broiled	3 oz cooked	54	197
	1 raw steak, edible portion = 3.2 oz	58	214
roasted	3 oz cooked	50	217
	1 raw steak, edible portion = 3.1 oz	52	225

SHORT LOIN, TOP
Lean & Fat

	Portion	Sodium (mg)	Calories
all grades, broiled	3 oz cooked	54	238
	1 raw steak, edible portion = 8.2 oz	148	651
choice, broiled	3 oz cooked	54	243
	1 raw steak, edible portion = 8.3 oz	148	672
good, broiled	3 oz cooked	54	223
	1 raw steak, edible portion = 8.1 oz	147	603
prime, broiled	3 oz cooked	53	288
	1 raw steak, edible portion = 8.1 oz	141	774

Lean Only

	Portion	Sodium (mg)	Calories
all grades, broiled	3 oz cooked	57	172
	1 raw steak, edible portion = 6.9 oz	132	395
choice, broiled	3 oz cooked	57	176
	1 raw steak, edible portion = 6.9 oz	133	406

	Portion	Sodium (mg)	Calories
good, broiled	3 oz cooked	57	162
	1 raw steak, edible portion = 6.9 oz	133	373
prime, broiled	3 oz cooked	57	208
	1 raw steak, edible portion = 6.3 oz	121	438

WEDGE-BONE SIRLOIN
Lean & Fat

all grades, broiled	3 oz cooked	53	238
	1 lb raw	177	791
choice			
broiled	3 oz cooked	53	240
	1 lb raw	177	804
pan-fried	3 oz cooked	58	288
	1 lb raw	184	913
good, broiled	3 oz cooked	53	232
	1 lb raw	177	777
prime, broiled	3 oz cooked	52	271
	1 lb raw	169	878

Lean Only

all grades, broiled	3 oz cooked	56	177
	1 lb raw	159	500
choice			
broiled	3 oz cooked	56	180
	1 lb raw	160	509
pan-fried	3 oz cooked	65	202
	1 lb raw	159	492
good, broiled	3 oz cooked	56	170
	1 lb raw	160	482
prime, broiled	3 oz cooked	56	201
	1 lb raw	148	527

VARIETY MEATS

brains			
pan-fried	3 oz cooked	134	167
	1 lb raw	555	690
simmered	3 oz cooked	102	136
	1 lb raw	469	627
heart, simmered	3 oz cooked	54	148
	1 lb raw	162	450
kidneys, simmered	3 oz cooked	114	122
	1 lb raw	264	283

	Portion	Sodium (mg)	Calories
liver			
braised	3 oz cooked	60	137
	1 lb raw	235	542
pan-fried	3 oz cooked	90	184
	1 lb raw	313	639
lungs, braised	3 oz cooked	86	102
	1 lb raw	306	365
tongue, simmered	3 oz cooked	51	241
	1 lb raw	155	732
tripe, raw	1 oz	13	28
	4 oz	52	111

Beef, Cured

	Portion	Sodium (mg)	Calories
breakfast strips, cooked	3 (15 per 12 oz pkg)	766	153
	6 oz	3,830	764
corned beef brisket, braised	3 oz cooked	964	213
	1 lb raw	3,628	802

▪ BRAND NAME

Oscar Mayer

	Portion	Sodium (mg)	Calories
breakfast strips, cooked	1 (15 per 12 oz pkg)	190	46

▫ BEVERAGES

See also FAST FOODS; MILK, MILK SUBSTITUTES, & MILK PRODUCTS

Beverages, Alcoholic

BEER & ALE

	Portion	Sodium (mg)	Calories
beer			
regular (4½% alcohol by volume)	12 fl oz	19	146
light (alcohol content of light beer varies)	12 fl oz	10	100

COCKTAILS & MIXED DRINKS

	Portion	Sodium (mg)	Calories
Bloody Mary	5 fl oz	332	116
bourbon & soda	4 fl oz	16	105
daiquiri cocktail	2 fl oz	3	111
daiquiri, canned	6.8 fl oz	12	
eggnog *See* Flavored Milk Beverages, *below*			

	Portion	Sodium (mg)	Calories
gin & tonic	7½ fl oz	10	171
manhattan	2 fl oz	2	128
martini	2½ fl oz	2	156
piña colada cocktail	4½ fl oz	9	262
piña colada, canned	6.8 fl oz	158	525
screwdriver	7 fl oz	2	174
tequila sunrise	5½ fl oz	7	189
tequila sunrise, canned	6.8 fl oz	119	
Tom Collins	7½ fl oz	39	121
whiskey sour cocktail	3 fl oz	10	123
whiskey sour mix			
bottled (no alcohol)	2 fl oz	66	55
prepared w/whiskey	2 fl oz mix + 1½ fl oz whiskey	66	158
powder	1 pkt	46	64
prepared w/water & whiskey	1 pkt + 1½ fl oz water + 1½ fl oz whiskey	48	169
whiskey sour, canned	6.8 fl oz	91	

CORDIALS & LIQUEURS

54 proof (22.1% alcohol by weight)	1 fl oz	1	97
coffee liqueur (53 proof)	1½ fl oz	4	174
coffee w/cream liqueur (34 proof)	1½ fl oz	43	154
crème de menthe liqueur (72 proof)	1½ fl oz	3	186

DISTILLED SPIRITS

all (gin, rum, vodka, whiskey)			
100 proof	1 fl oz	0	82
	1½ fl oz	0	124
94 proof	1 fl oz	0	76
	1½ fl oz	0	116
gin, 90 proof	1½ fl oz	1	110
rum, 80 proof	1½ fl oz	0	97
vodka, 80 proof	1½ fl oz	0	97
whiskey, 86 proof	1½ fl oz	0	105

WINES

dessert wine, sweet, 18.8% alcohol by volume	1 fl oz	3	46
muscatel or port	3½ fl oz	4	158
sherry	2 fl oz	2	84
table wine, 11½% alcohol by volume			
red	1 fl oz	2	21
	3½ fl oz	6	74

	Portion	Sodium (mg)	Calories
table wine *(cont.)*			
rosé	1 fl oz	1	21
	3½ fl oz	5	73
white	1 fl oz	2	20
	3½ fl oz	5	70
vermouth, dry, French	3½ fl oz	4	105

Beverages, Carbonated

	Portion	Sodium (mg)	Calories
bitter lemon	12 fl oz	60	192
club soda	12 fl oz	75	0
cola	12 fl oz	14	151
low-cal, aspartame-sweetened	12 fl oz	21	2
low-cal, sodium-saccharin-sweetened	12 fl oz	57	2
cream soda	12 fl oz	43	191
ginger ale	12 fl oz	25	124
grape soda	12 fl oz	57	161
lemon-lime soda	12 fl oz	41	149
orange soda	12 fl oz	46	177
peach soda	12 fl oz	33	184
quinine water	4 fl oz	8	37
root beer	12 fl oz	49	152
diet	12 fl oz	59	1
strawberry soda	12 fl oz	14	174
tonic water	12 fl oz	15	125

Coffee & Coffee Substitutes

	Portion	Sodium (mg)	Calories
coffee substitute, cereal grain beverage, powder			
prepared w/water	6 fl oz water + 1 t powder	7	9
prepared w/whole milk	6 fl oz milk + 1 t powder	91	121
coffee, brewed	6 fl oz	4	4
coffee, instant, regular or de-caffeinated, powder, prepared w/water	6 fl oz water + 1 rounded t powder	6	4

Flavored Milk Beverages

	Portion	Sodium (mg)	Calories
carob-flavored mix			
powder	3 t	12	45
powder, prepared w/whole milk	1 c milk + 3 t powder	132	195
chocolate dairy drink, reduced-calorie, aspartame-sweet-ened, powder, prepared w/water	½ c water + 3 ice cubes + ¾ oz pkt	172	64

	Portion	Sodium (mg)	Calories
chocolate-flavored mix			
powder	2–3 heaping t	45	75
powder, prepared w/whole milk	1 c milk + 2–3 heaping t powder	165	226
chocolate milk			
whole	1 c	149	208
low-fat, 2%	1 c	150	179
low-fat, 1%	1 c	152	158
chocolate syrup			
w/added nutrients	1 T	29	46
prepared w/whole milk	1 c milk + 1 T syrup	148	196
w/out added nutrients	1 fl oz	36	82
prepared w/whole milk	1 c milk + 2 T syrup	156	232
cocoa, homemade, w/whole milk	6 fl oz	92	164
	1 c	123	218
cocoa mix			
reduced-calorie, aspartame-sweetened, powder, prepared w/water	6 fl oz water + .53 oz pkt	173	48
w/added nutrients	6 fl oz water + 1 pkt	207	120
w/out added nutrients	6 fl oz water + 3–4 heaping t powder	149	103
eggnog, dairy	1 c	138	342
eggnog-flavored mix, powder, prepared w/whole milk	1 c milk + 2 heaping t powder	163	260
malted milk–flavored mix, chocolate			
w/added nutrients			
powder	¾ oz or 4–5 heaping t	125	75
powder, prepared w/whole milk	1 c milk + 4–5 heaping t powder	244	225
w/out added nutrients			
powder	¾ oz or 3 heaping t	53	79
powder, prepared w/whole milk	1 c milk + 3 heaping t powder	172	229

	Portion	Sodium (mg)	Calories
malted milk–flavored mix, natural			
w/added nutrients			
powder	¾ oz or 4–5 heaping t	85	80
powder, prepared w/whole milk	1 c milk + 4–5 heaping t powder	205	230
w/out added nutrients			
powder	¾ oz or 3 heaping t	103	87
powder, prepared w/whole milk	1 c milk + 3 heaping t powder	223	237
shake, thick			
chocolate	10 oz	314	335
	10.6 oz	333	356
vanilla	10 oz	270	315
	about 11 oz	299	350
strawberry-flavored mix, powder, prepared w/whole milk	1 c milk + 2–3 heaping t powder	128	234

Fruit & Vegetable Juices

	Portion	Sodium (mg)	Calories
acerola	1 c	7	51
apple			
canned or bottled	1 c	7	116
from frozen concentrate	1 c	17	111
apricot, canned	1 c	9	141
carrot, canned	½ c	36	49
cranberry, bottled	1 c	10	147
grape			
canned	1 c	7	155
from frozen concentrate, sweetened	1 c	5	128
grapefruit			
fresh	1 c	2	96
canned			
sweetened	1 c	4	116
unsweetened	1 c	3	93
from frozen concentrate	1 c	2	102
lemon, canned or bottled	1 T	3	3
lime, canned or bottled	1 T	2	3
orange			
fresh	1 c	2	111
canned	1 c	6	104
from frozen concentrate	1 c	2	112
frozen concentrate, undiluted	6 fl oz	7	339

	Portion	Sodium (mg)	Calories
orange-grapefruit, canned	1 c	8	107
papaya, canned	1 c	14	142
passion fruit, yellow	1 c	15	149
peach, canned	1 c	17	134
pear, canned	1 c	9	149
pineapple			
canned	1 c	2	139
from frozen concentrate	1 c	3	129
prune, canned	1 c	11	181
tangerine			
canned, sweetened	1 c	2	125
fresh	1 c	2	106
from frozen concentrate, sweetened	1 c	2	110
tomato, canned	6 fl oz	658	32
w/beef broth	5½ fl oz	220	61
w/clam juice	5½ fl oz	604	77
vegetable, canned	6 fl oz	664	34

Fruit Juice Drinks (10–50% Fruit Juice), Juice Ades, & Juice-flavored Drinks & Powders

	Portion	Sodium (mg)	Calories
apple juice drink, canned	6 fl oz	12	92
cherry juice drink, canned	6 fl oz	4	93
citrus fruit drink, canned	6 fl oz	4	93
citrus fruit juice drink, from frozen concentrate	1 c	7	114
cranberry juice cocktail			
bottled	6 fl oz	4	108
from frozen concentrate	6 fl oz	6	102
low-cal, calcium-saccharin- & corn-sweetened, bottled	6 fl oz	6	33
cranberry-apple juice drink, bottled	6 fl oz	4	123
cranberry-apricot juice drink, bottled	6 fl oz	4	118
cranberry-grape juice drink, bottled	6 fl oz	5	103
Florida punch juice drink, canned	6 fl oz	35	95
fruit punch drink			
canned	6 fl oz	41	87
from frozen concentrate	1 c	11	113
fruit punch juice drink, from frozen concentrate	1 c	12	123
fruit punch–flavored drink, powder, prepared w/water	1 c water + 2 rounded T powder	38	97
gelatin drink, orange-flavored, powder	0.6 oz pkt	29	67

	Portion	Sodium (mg)	Calories
grape drink, canned	6 fl oz	12	84
grape juice drink, canned	6 fl oz	2	94
lemon-lime, from mix	8 fl oz	30	91
lemonade			
from frozen concentrate	1 c	8	100
powder, low-cal, aspartame-sweetened	0.42 oz pkt	1	40
	0.67 oz pkt	2	63
powder, prepared w/water	1 c water + 2 T powder	13	102
lemonade-flavored drink, powder, prepared w/water	1 c water + 2 T powder	19	113
limeade, from frozen concentrate	1 c	6	102
orange drink, breakfast type, from frozen concentrate (orange juice & orange pulp)	6 fl oz	18	84
orange drink, canned	6 fl oz	31	94
orange juice drink, canned	6 fl oz	58	92
orange-flavored drink, breakfast type			
from frozen concentrate w/orange pulp	6 fl oz	17	91
from powder	3 rounded t powder + 6 fl oz water	9	86
orange-pineapple juice drink, canned	6 fl oz	1	94
peach juice drink, canned	6 fl oz	tr	90
pineapple & grapefruit juice drink, canned	1 c	34	117
pineapple & orange juice drink, canned	1 c	9	125
pineapple-orange juice drink, canned	6 fl oz	6	99
strawberry juice drink, canned	6 fl oz	tr	89
tangerine juice drink, canned	6 fl oz	tr	90
wild berry juice drink, canned	6 fl oz	5	88

Tea

	Portion	Sodium (mg)	Calories
brewed	6 fl oz	5	2
herb, brewed	6 fl oz	2	1
instant, powder			
low-cal, sodium-saccharin-sweetened, lemon-flavored	2 t	17	5
sweetened	3 t in 8 fl oz water	49	86
unsweetened	1 t	1	2
unsweetened, lemon-flavored	1 rounded t	7	4

	Portion	Sodium (mg)	Calories

Water

municipal (mineral content will vary depending on water source)	1 c	7	0

▪ BRAND NAME

7-Up

Cherry 7-Up	6 oz	0	74
Diet 7-Up	6 oz	16	2
Diet 7-Up Gold	6 oz	16	<2
Diet Cherry 7-Up	6 oz	4	2
7-Up	6 oz	16	72
7-Up Gold	6 oz	8	13

Apple & Eve Juices

apple	6 fl oz	3	75
apple cider	6 fl oz	8	83
apple cranberry	6 fl oz	5	75
apple grape	6 fl oz	3	83
cranberry-grape	6 fl oz	4	94
raspberry-cranberry	6 fl oz	9	86

Awake

from frozen concentrate	6 fl oz	15	91

Campbell Juices

apple	6 oz	50	110
grape	6 oz	50	110
grapefruit	6 oz	20	80
orange	6 oz	40	90
tomato	6 oz	570	35

Coca-Cola Soft Drinks

Caffeine-Free	6 fl oz	4	77
Caffeine-Free Diet Coke	6 fl oz	4	1
Caffeine-Free Tab	6 fl oz	4	tr
cherry	6 fl oz	4	76
Classic	6 fl oz	7	72
Coca-Cola	6 fl oz	4	77
diet cherry	6 fl oz	4	1
Diet Coke	6 fl oz	4	1
Diet Sprite	6 fl oz	tr	0
Fresca	6 fl oz	tr	2
Mello Yello	6 fl oz	14	87
Mr. Pibb	12 fl oz	10	143
Ramblin' Root Beer	6 fl oz	17	88
Sprite	6 fl oz	23	71
Tab	6 fl oz	4	tr

	Portion	Sodium (mg)	Calories
Country Time Drink Mix			
lemon-lime, sugar-sweetened	8 fl oz	20	80
lemonade & pink lemonade			
sugar-sweetened	8 fl oz	20	80
w/NutraSweet	8 fl oz	0	4
Crystal Light Drink Mix			
all	8 fl oz	0	4
Dole Juices			
New pineapple	6 oz	7	100
New pineapple-grapefruit	6 oz	8	90
New pineapple-orange	6 oz	8	100
pineapple	6 oz	2	103
pineapple–pink grapefruit	6 oz	tr	101
Dr. Pepper Soft Drinks			
Caffeine-Free Pepper Free	6 fl oz	9	72
Diet Dr. Pepper	6 fl oz	9	1
Diet Pepper Free	6 fl oz	9	1
Dr. Pepper	6 fl oz	9	72
Fanta Soft Drinks			
ginger ale	6 fl oz	14	63
grape	6 fl oz	7	86
orange	6 fl oz	7	88
root beer	6 fl oz	10	78
Featherweight			
hot cocoa, low-cal	.44 oz	110	50
tomato juice, low-sodium	6 oz	10	35
Five Alive Fruit Drinks			
CARTONS			
berry citrus	6 fl oz	15	123
citrus	6 fl oz	16	122
tropical citrus	6 fl oz	15	123
FROZEN CONCENTRATE			
berry citrus	6 fl oz	1	88
citrus	6 fl oz	2	87
tropical citrus	6 fl oz	1	85
Gatorade			
lemon-lime or orange flavor, w/water	8 fl oz	110	50
Hawaiian Punch			
Fruit Juicy Red			
regular	6 fl oz	20	90
light	6 fl oz	30	60

	Portion	Sodium (mg)	Calories
grape	6 fl oz	30	90
Island Fruit Cocktail	6 fl oz	30	90
orange	6 fl oz	20	100
tropical fruit	6 fl oz	30	90
Very Berry	6 fl oz	30	90
Wild Fruit	6 fl oz	35	90
Hershey			
chocolate-flavored syrup	2 T	20	80
chocolate milk, 2% low-fat	1 c	130	190
cocoa	⅓ c	10	120
instant cocoa	3 T	45	80
Hi-C Fruit Drinks			
Candy Apple Cooler	8.45 fl oz	25	132
Double Fruit Cooler	8.45 fl oz	25	131
fruit punch	8.45 fl oz	24	135
grape	8.45 fl oz	24	136
Hula punch	8.45 fl oz	24	122
lemonade	8.45 fl oz	24	109
orange	8.45 fl oz	24	134
Wild Berry	8.45 fl oz	24	129
International Coffees _SUGAR-FREE_			
Cafe Amaretto	6 fl oz	20	35
Cafe Français	6 fl oz	20	35
Cafe Irish Creme	6 fl oz	15	30
Cafe Vienna	6 fl oz	95	30
Irish Mocha Mint	6 fl oz	20	25
Orange Cappuccino	6 fl oz	60	30
Suisse Mocha	6 fl oz	20	30
SWEETENED W/SUGAR			
Cafe Amaretto	6 fl oz	25	50
Cafe Français	6 fl oz	25	50
Cafe Irish Creme	6 fl oz	20	60
Cafe Vienna	6 fl oz	105	60
Double Dutch Chocolate	6 fl oz	15	50
Irish Mocha Mint	6 fl oz	20	50
Orange Cappuccino	6 fl oz	105	60
Suisse Mocha	6 fl oz	25	50
Kool-Aid _KOOLERS_			
all	8.45 fl oz	10	130
SOFT DRINK MIX			
Sugar-free			
grape	8 fl oz	0	4

	Portion	Sodium (mg)	Calories
Mountain Berry punch	8 fl oz	35	4
Rainbow punch	8 fl oz	0	4
Tropical punch	8 fl oz	10	4
Sugar-sweetened			
grape	8 fl oz	25	80
Rainbow punch	8 fl oz	20	80
Tropical punch	8 fl oz	0	80
Unsweetened, Prepared w/Sugar			
Rainbow punch	8 fl oz	0	100
Sunshine punch	8 fl oz	0	100
Tropical punch	8 fl oz	10	100
Light 'n Juicy Juice Drinks			
grape, carton	6 fl oz	17	13
lemonade, carton	6 fl oz	17	8
orange, carton	6 fl oz	17	16
punch, carton	6 fl oz	17	14
Like Cola			
Like Cola	6 oz	3	12–13
Sugar-Free Like Cola	6 oz	11	<1
Minute Maid			
FRUIT ADES			
Country Style lemonade			
carton	6 fl oz	23	81
from frozen concentrate	6 fl oz	23	72
grapeade, carton or from frozen concentrate	6 fl oz	18	94
lemonade or pink lemonade			
carton	6 fl oz	23	81
from frozen concentrate	6 fl oz	23	77
FRUIT JUICES			
apple, carton or from frozen concentrate	6 fl oz	23	91
citrus punch			
carton	6 fl oz	17	94
from frozen concentrate	6 fl oz	17	92
grape, sweetened, from frozen concentrate	6 fl oz	21	100
grapefruit			
carton	6 fl oz	19	78
from frozen concentrate	6 fl oz	19	83
grapefruit, pink, from frozen concentrate	6 fl oz	19	78
lemon juice, from frozen concentrate	1 T	2	4

	Portion	Sodium (mg)	Calories
orange			
regular, carton or from frozen concentrate	6 fl oz	19	91
calcium-fortified, carton or from frozen concentrate	6 fl oz	19	93
Country Style, carton or from frozen concentrate	6 fl oz	19	91
pineapple orange, from frozen concentrate	6 fl oz	19	98
pineapple, from frozen concentrate	6 fl oz	19	99
tangerine, sweetened, from frozen concentrate	6 fl oz	19	91

SOFT DRINKS

diet lemon-lime	6 fl oz	1	10
diet orange	6 fl oz	tr	8
lemon-lime	6 fl oz	1	71
orange	6 fl oz	tr	87

Mott's
JUICE DRINKS

apple cranberry drink	10 oz	3	176
apple raspberry drink	10 oz	17	158
Beefamato	6 oz	240	80
Clamato	6 oz	815	96
fruit punch	10 oz	4	170
grape apple drink	10 oz	tr	167
orange fruit juice blend	10 oz	6	144

JUICES

apple	6 oz	13	88
apple cranberry	6 oz	17	83
apple grape	6 oz	17	86
apple raspberry	6 oz	48	83
apple, natural	6 oz	28	76
grapefruit	10 oz	5	124
prune			
regular	6 oz	8	130
Country Style	6 oz	7	130

Ocean Spray

apple juice	6 fl oz	14	90
Cran-Blueberry	6 fl oz	10	120
Cran-Grape	6 fl oz	5	130
Cran-Raspberry	6 fl oz	10	110
Cran-Tastic	6 fl oz	15	110
Cranapple	6 fl oz	10	130
Cranberry Juice Cocktail	6 fl oz	10	110
Cranicot	6 fl oz	5	110

	Portion	Sodium (mg)	Calories
grapefruit juice	6 fl oz	10	70
Low-Calorie Cran-Raspberry	6 fl oz	10	40
Low-Calorie Cranapple	6 fl oz	10	40
Low-Calorie Cranberry Juice Cocktail	6 fl oz	10	40
Mauna La'i Hawaiian Guava Fruit Drink	6 fl oz	10	100
Mauna La'i Hawaiian Guava Passion Fruit Drink	6 fl oz	15	100
Pink Grapefruit Juice Cocktail	6 fl oz	10	80
Orange Plus			
from frozen concentrate	6 fl oz	9	97
Ortega			
Snap-E-Tom tomato cocktail	6 fl oz	750	40
Ovaltine Drink Mixes			
chocolate	¾ oz dry mix	145	80
	¾ oz dry mix + 8 oz 2% milk	270	200
cocoa			
50-calorie	0.45 oz or about 2½ t	150	50
Hot 'n Rich	1 oz or 5 t	170	120
sugar-free	0.41 oz or about 2½ t	160	40
malt	¾ oz dry mix	56	80
	¾ oz dry mix + 8 oz 2% milk	178	200
Pepsi			
Diet Lemon-Lime Slice	12 oz	11	26
Diet Mandarin Orange Slice	12 oz	41	19
Diet Pepsi	12 oz	54	1
Diet Pepsi Free	12 oz	70	1
Lemon-Lime Slice	12 oz	11	152
Mandarin Orange Slice	12 oz	22	193
Mountain Dew	12 fl oz	31	178
Pepsi-Cola	12 fl oz	10	157
Pepsi Free	12 oz	13	157
Perrier			
water, bottled	8 fl oz	3	0
Poland Spring			
water, bottled	1 c	1	0
Postum			
instant hot beverage, regular or coffee-flavored	6 fl oz	0	12

	Portion	Sodium (mg)	Calories
Rose Holland			
JUICE-FLAVORED DRINKS			
grenadine	1 fl oz	27	65
lime juice	1 fl oz	6	48
LIQUID DRINK MIXES			
Coco Casa			
cream of coconut	1 fl oz	21	81
piña colada	1 fl oz	107	33
daiquiri	1 fl oz	111	36
mai tai	1 fl oz	60	32
manhattan	1 fl oz	5	28
margarita	1 fl oz	92	27
old fashioned	1 fl oz	6	33
piña colada	1 fl oz	4	33
Smooth & Spicy Bloody Mary	1 fl oz	329	3
strawberry daiquiri	1 fl oz	3	31
strawberry margarita	1 fl oz	3	31
sweet & sour	1 fl oz	107	34
Tom Collins	1 fl oz	96	47
whiskey sour	1 fl oz	105	37
Royal Crown			
Diet RC 100	12 fl oz	1	2
RC 100	12 fl oz	1	156
RC Cola	12 fl oz	1	156
Schweppes			
bitter lemon	6 oz	13	82
club soda	6 oz	25	tr
Collins mixer	6 oz	51	75
diet ginger ale	6 oz	39	<2
diet tonic water	6 oz	45	<2
ginger ale	6 oz	30	70
ginger beer	6 oz	30	70
grape soda	6 oz	15	95
grapefruit	6 oz	28	80
lemon lime	6 oz	30	72
lemon sour	6 oz	12	79
root beer	6 oz	17	76
seltzer water (sodium-free)	6 oz	<5	0
sparkling orange	6 oz	17	88
tonic water	6 oz	8	64
Vichy water	6 oz	76	tr
Sprite			
soda	12 fl oz	46	142
Sunrise			
flavored instant coffee	0.07 oz + 6 fl oz water	5	6

	Portion	Sodium (mg)	Calories
Tang			
breakfast beverage crystals, average of grape, grapefruit, & orange			
regular	6 fl oz	0	90
sugar-free	6 fl oz	0	6
grape	3 rounded t in 6 fl oz water	0	89
grapefruit	3 rounded t in 6 fl oz water	0	87
orange	3 rounded t in 6 fl oz water	0	89
V8			
Spicy Hot V8	6 oz	600	35
vegetable juice			
regular	6 oz	600	35
no salt added	6 oz	45	40

❏ **BISCUITS** *See* **BREADS, ROLLS, BISCUITS, & MUFFINS**

❏ **BREADCRUMBS, CROUTONS, STUFFINGS, & SEASONED COATINGS**

	Portion	Sodium (mg)	Calories
breadcrumbs			
enriched, dry, grated	1 c	736	390
white bread, enriched, soft	1 c	231	120
bread cubes, white, enriched	1 c	154	80
cornflake crumbs	1 oz	305	110
croutons, herb-seasoned	0.7 oz	260	70
stuffing, from mix			
bread	½ c	504	208
corn bread	½ c	434	117
enriched bread			
moist type	1 c	1,023	420
dry type	1 c	1,254	500

• **BRAND NAME**

	Portion	Sodium (mg)	Calories
Arnold Croutons			
Cheddar Romano Crispy	½ oz	154	64
Cheese Garlic Crispy	½ oz	133	60

	Portion	Sodium (mg)	Calories
Fine Herbs Crispy	½ oz	151	53
Italian Crispy	½ oz	148	62
Seasoned Crispy	½ oz	161	60
Devonsheer Breadcrumbs			
plain	1 oz	272	108
Italian Style	1 oz	408	104
Kellogg's			
cornflake crumbs	1 oz	290	110
Croutettes	0.7 oz dry	260	70
Nabisco			
cracker meal	2 T	0	50
Pepperidge Farm			
croutons	½ c	160–220	70
stuffings	1 oz	210–330	110
CROUTONS			
cheese & garlic	½ oz	180	70
onion & garlic	½ oz	160	70
seasoned	½ oz	210	70
STUFFINGS			
corn bread	1 oz	320	110
cube	1 oz	430	110
herb-seasoned	1 oz	410	110
Pillsbury Stuffing Originals			
chicken	½ c	670	170
corn bread	½ c	660	170
mushroom	½ c	780	150
wild rice	½ c	540	160
Rice-A-Roni Stuffing Mixes			
bread w/wild rice, prepared	½ c	750	240
bread/chicken flavor w/rice, prepared	½ c	780	240
bread/herb & butter & wild rice, prepared	½ c	850	240
corn bread w/rice, prepared	½ c	910	240
Shake 'n Bake Seasoned Coatings			
Country Mild Recipe	¼ pouch	500	80
Extra Crispy			
for chicken	¼ pouch	810	110
for pork	¼ pouch	690	120
Homestyle for chicken	¼ pouch	950	80

	Portion	Sodium (mg)	Calories
Stove Top			
FLEXIBLE SERVING STUFFING MIX			
chicken flavor, w/salted butter	½ c	570	170
corn bread flavor, w/salted butter	½ c	590	170
Homestyle herb, w/salted butter	½ c	530	170
STUFFING MIX			
Americana New England, w/ salted butter	½ c	630	180
Americana San Francisco, w/ salted butter	½ c	640	170
beef, w/salted butter	½ c	580	180
chicken flavor, w/salted butter	½ c	560	180
corn bread, w/salted butter	½ c	570	170
long grain & wild rice, w/salted butter	½ c	550	180
savory herbs, w/salted butter	½ c	580	180
turkey, w/salted butter	½ c	630	170
wild rice, w/salted butter	½ c	550	180

❑ BREADS, ROLLS, BISCUITS, & MUFFINS

Biscuits

	Portion	Sodium (mg)	Calories
baking powder, prepared w/ vegetable shortening			
from mix	1 (2″ diam)	262	95
from refrigerator dough	1 (2″ diam)	249	65
homemade	1 (2″ diam)	175	100
buttermilk, from refrigerator dough	2	410	130
flaky, from refrigerator dough	2	580	180

Bread & Bread Sticks

	Portion	Sodium (mg)	Calories
Boston brown bread, canned	1.6 oz slice	113	95
bread sticks			
regular	1	100	23
Vienna	1	94	18
coffee cake *See* DESSERTS: CAKES, PASTRIES, & PIES			
corn bread			
from mix	1 piece	263	178
homemade			
w/enriched cornmeal	2.9 oz	232	198
w/whole-ground cornmeal	2.7 oz	209	172

	Portion	Sodium (mg)	Calories
cracked-wheat bread	1 lb loaf	1,966	1,190
	0.9 oz slice	106	65
danish *See* DESSERTS: CAKES, PASTRIES, & PIES			
French bread	1 lb loaf	2,633	1,270
	1.2 oz slice	203	100
fruit & nut quick bread, from mix	1.4 oz slice	126	118
honey wheatberry bread	1 oz slice	161	70
Italian bread	1 lb loaf	2,656	1,255
	1 oz slice	176	85
matzo *See* CRACKERS			
mixed-grain bread	1 lb loaf	1,870	1,165
	0.9 oz slice	106	65
oatmeal bread	1 lb loaf	2,231	1,145
	0.9 oz slice	124	65
pita bread, white	1 piece (6½″ diam)	339	165
pumpernickel bread	1 lb loaf	2,461	1,160
	1.1 oz slice	177	80
raisin bread	1 lb loaf	1,657	1,260
	0.9 oz slice	92	65
roman meal bread	1 oz slice	140	70
rye bread, light	1 lb loaf	3,164	1,190
	0.9 oz slice	175	65
sourdough bread	1 oz slice	154	68
Vienna bread	1 lb loaf	2,633	1,270
	0.9 oz slice	145	70
wheat bread	1 lh loaf	2,447	1,160
	0.9 oz slice	138	65
wheatberry bread	1 oz slice	148	70
white bread	1 lb loaf	2,334	1,210
	0.9 oz slice	129	65
white bread	0.7 oz slice	101	55
whole-wheat bread	1 lb loaf	2,887	1,110
	1 oz slice	180	70

Muffins

	Portion	Sodium (mg)	Calories
blueberry			
from mix	1.6 oz	225	140
homemade	1.6 oz	198	135
bran			
from mix	1.6 oz	385	140
homemade	1.6 oz	169	125
corn			
from mix	1.6 oz	450	145
homemade	1.6 oz	169	145
English			
regular	2 oz	378	140
sourdough	2 oz	252	129

	Portion	Sodium (mg)	Calories
Rolls & Bagels			
bagel			
plain or water, enriched	1 (3½″ diam)	245	200
brown & serve roll	1	157	92
butterflake roll, from refrigerator dough	1	445	110
buttermilk roll, from mix	1	343	113
crescent roll, from refrigerator dough	2	665	200
croissant	2 oz	452	235
dinner roll			
commercial	1 oz	155	85
homemade	1.2 oz	98	120
frankfurter or hamburger roll	1.4 oz	241	115
French roll, enriched	1 = 1.8 oz	287	137
hard roll, commercial	1.2 oz	313	155
hoagie or submarine roll	4.8 oz	683	400
parkerhouse roll	0.6 oz	105	59
popover, homemade	1	88	90
raisin roll	2.1 oz	230	165
rye roll	0.6 oz	120	55
dark, hard	1 oz	254	80
light, hard	1 oz	247	79
sandwich roll	1.8 oz	335	162
sesame seed roll	0.6 oz	105	59
sweet roll *See* DESSERTS: CAKES, PASTRIES, & PIES			
wheat roll	0.6 oz	126	52
white roll			
from mix	2.2 oz	255	190
from refrigerator dough	1 oz	335	90
homemade	1.2 oz	98	119
whole-wheat roll, homemade	1.2 oz	197	90
Tortillas			
taco/tostada shell, corn	0.4 oz	72	50
tortilla, corn	1.1 oz	1	65
canned	1.2 oz	191	75
▪ BRAND NAME			
Arnold			
BREADS			
Bakery Light Golden Wheat	1 slice	86	44
Bakery Light Italian	1 slice	90	45
Bakery Light Oatmeal	1 slice	98	44

	Portion	Sodium (mg)	Calories
Bran'nola County Oat	1 slice	166	90
Bran'nola Dark Wheat	1 slice	166	83
Bran'nola Hearty Wheat	1 slice	197	88
Bran'nola Nutty Grains	1 slice	144	85
Bran'nola Original	1 slice	137	85
Brick Oven Extra Fiber White	1 slice	93	55
Brick Oven White	1 slice	163	79
Brown Natural Wheat	1 slice	183	80
cinnamon raisin	1 slice	86	67
Country White	1 slice	204	98
dill rye	1 slice	187	71
Francisco International Italian Thick Sliced	1 slice	111	66
honey wheatberry	1 slice	143	77
Jewish rye			
w/out seeds	1 slice	167	71
w/seeds	1 slice	170	70
melba thin rye	1 slice	112	44
#1 Brick Oven Wheat	1 slice	194	60
orange raisin	1 slice	85	67
pumpernickel	1 slice	198	70
stoneground 100% whole wheat	1 slice	97	48

ROLLS

Dinner Party roll	1	81	51
Dutch egg sandwich bun	1	203	123
hamburger bun	1	223	115
soft sandwich roll	1	194	110

Lender's Bagels

blueberry	1	250	190
egg	1	360	150
garlic	1	340	160
onion	1	290	160
plain	1	320	150
poppy seed	1	370	160
pumpernickel	1	330	160
rye	1	310	150
sesame seed	1	320	160
Wheat 'n Raisin	1	310	190

Levy's Jewish Rye

w/out seeds	1 slice	178	75
w/seeds	1 slice	181	76

Ortega

taco/tostada shells	1	5	50

Pepperidge Farm
BREADS

Cinnamon Swirl	2 slices	196	160
cracked-wheat	2 slices	280	130

	Portion	Sodium (mg)	Calories
Dijon rye	2 slices	340	100
honey bran	2 slices	340	180
honey wheatberry	2 slices	290	130
large Family white	2 slices	290	150
multigrain, very thin	2 slices	180	80
oatmeal	2 slices	370	130
Party Dijon Slices	4 slices	170	70
Party Pumpernickel Slices	4 slices	180	70
Party Rye Slices	4 slices	280	60
raisin w/cinnamon	2 slices	170	140
Sandwich White	2 slices	270	130
seeded Family rye	2 slices	430	160
seedless rye	2 slices	420	150
Toasting White	2 slices	430	130
wheat	2 slices	380	180
wheat germ	2 slices	280	120
white, very thin	2 slices	150	60
whole-wheat	2 slices	250	120
whole-wheat, very thin	2 slices	150	60

ENGLISH MUFFINS

plain	1	200	140
cinnamon raisin	1	180	150

OLD FASHIONED MUFFINS, FROZEN

blueberry	1	250	180
bran w/raisins	1	300	180
carrot walnut	1	222	170
cinnamon swirl	1	170	190
corn	1	260	180

ROLLS

butter crescent	1	150	110
club, brown & serve	1	200	100
French style	1	230	110
golden twist	1	150	110
hamburger	1	240	130
onion sandwich buns w/poppy seeds	1	260	150
parkerhouse	1	80	60
sourdough-style French	1	240	100

Pillsbury
BISCUITS

Big Country Southern Style	2	650	200
buttermilk	2	360	100
Country	2	360	100
Extra Lights flaky buttermilk	2	340	110
Hungry Jack			
buttermilk fluffy	2	560	180
extra-rich buttermilk	2	340	100
flaky	2	600	160

	Portion	Sodium (mg)	Calories
Tenderflake baking powder dinner	2	340	110
BREAD STICKS			
soft	1	230	100
DINNER ROLLS			
butterflake	1	520	140
crescent	2	460	200
PIPIN' HOT BREADS			
Crusty French	1" slice	120	60
wheat	1" slice	170	80
white	1" slice	170	80

SWEET ROLLS & TURNOVERS See DESSERTS: CAKES, PASTRIES, & PIES

	Portion	Sodium (mg)	Calories
Sahara Pita Bread			
wheat	1 miniloaf	155	66
white	1 miniloaf or ½ regular loaf	147	79
Sara Lee			
BAGELS			
cinnamon & raisin	1	280	240
egg	1	410	240
onion	1	630	220
plain	1	540	230
poppy seed	1	580	230
sesame seed	1	570	260
HEARTY FRUIT MUFFINS			
apple cinnamon spice	1	280	220
blueberry	1	330	200
Golden Corn	1	330	250
oat bran	1	380	220
raisin bran	1	400	220
L'ORIGINAL CROISSANTS			
all butter	1	240	170
petite size	1	160	120
cheese & broccoli	1	600	340
ham & Swiss cheese	1	860	340
Thomas's			
BREADS			
Fiber Calcium	1 slice	91	52
Lite Wheat	1 slice	72	41

	Portion	Sodium (mg)	Calories
ENGLISH MUFFINS			
regular	1	206	130
honey wheat	1	199	128
raisin, w/cinnamon	1	183	151

❑ BREAKFAST CEREALS, COLD & HOT

Cold Cereal

	Portion	Sodium (mg)	Calories
cornflakes, low-sodium	1 oz or about 1 c	3	113
crisp rice			
regular	1 oz or about 1 c	208	112
low-sodium	1 oz or about 1 c	3	114
granola, homemade	1 oz or about ¼ c	3	138
	1 c	12	595
honey bran	1 oz or about ⅞ c	164	97
	1 c	202	119
oat flakes, fortified	1 oz or about ⅔ c	253	105
	1 c	429	177
raisins, rice & rye	1.3 oz or about 1 c	280	124
rice, puffed	½ oz or about 1 c	0	57
sugar-sparkled flakes	1 oz box	160	109
wheat germ, toasted			
plain	1 oz or about ¼ c	1	108
	1 c	4	431
w/brown sugar & honey	1 oz or about ¼ c	1	107
	1 c	3	426
wheat, puffed, plain	½ oz or about 1 c (heaping)	49	52
wheat, shredded			
large biscuit	1 rectangular	0	83
	2 round	1	133
small biscuit	1 oz or about ⅔ c	3	102
	⅞ oz box	3	89

	Portion	Sodium (mg)	Calories
Hot Cereal			
corn grits			
regular & quick			
dry	1 c	1	579
	1 T	0	36
cooked	1 c	0	146
	¾ c	0	110
instant, prepared			
plain	1 pkt	344	82
w/artificial cheese flavor	1 pkt	481	107
w/imitation bacon bits	1 pkt	531	104
w/imitation ham bits	1 pkt	657	103
farina			
dry	1 c	5	649
	1 T	0	40
cooked	1 c	1	110
	¾ c	1	87
grits; hominy grits *See* corn grits, *above*			
oats, regular, quick, & instant, nonfortified			
dry	⅓ c	1	104
cooked	1 c	1	145
	¾ c	1	108
▪ **BRAND NAME**			
Arrowhead Mills			
COLD CEREAL			
Agrain & Agrain	2 oz	2	220
Arrowhead Crunch	1 oz	40	120
bran flakes	1 oz	4	100
corn, puffed	½ oz	1	50
cornflakes	1 oz	15	110
granola			
apple amaranth	2 oz	3	225
maple nut	2 oz	25	260
millet, puffed	½ oz	1	50
Nature O's	1 oz	tr	110
rice, puffed	½ oz	1	50
wheat bran	2 oz	5	200
wheat germ, raw	2 oz	2	210
wheat, puffed	½ oz	1	50
HOT CEREAL			
Bear Mush	1 oz	1	100
corn grits			
white	2 oz	1	200
yellow	2 oz	1	200
4 Grain & Flax	2 oz	1	94

	Portion	Sodium (mg)	Calories
oat bran	1 oz	2	110
oatmeal, instant	1 oz	0	100
oats, steel cut	2 oz	1	220
Rice & Shine	¼ c	1	160
Seven Grain	1 oz	1	100
wheat, cracked	2 oz	2	180
Erewhon			
COLD CEREAL			
Crispy Brown Rice			
regular	1 oz or about 1 c	185	110
low-sodium	1 oz or about 1 c	tr	110
Fruit 'n Wheat	1 oz or about ½ c	8	100
granola			
date nut	1 oz or about ¼ c	45	130
honey almond	1 oz or about ¼ c	65	130
maple	1 oz or about ¼ c	55	130
#9, w/bran, no salt added	1 oz or about ¼ c	1	130
spiced apple	1 oz or about ¼ c	55	130
Sunflower Crunch	1 oz or about ¼ c	60	130
raisin bran	1 oz or about ½ c	80	100
wheat flakes	1 oz or about ½ c	75	110
HOT CEREAL			
Barley Plus	1 oz or about ⅓ c dry	0	110
brown rice cream	1 oz or about ⅓ c dry	20	110
oat bran w/toasted wheat germ	1 oz or about ⅓ c dry	15	115
Featherweight Cold Cereal			
cornflakes	1¼ c	<10	110
General Mills Cold Cereal			
Cheerios			
regular	1 oz or about 1¼ c	307	111
	¾ oz box	231	83
Honey Nut	1 oz or about ¾ c	257	107
	1 c	299	125

	Portion	Sodium (mg)	Calories
Crispy Wheats 'n Raisins	1 oz or about ¾ c	135	99
	1 c	204	150
Golden Grahams	1 oz or about ¾ c	346	109
	1 c	476	150
Kix	1 oz or about 1½ c	339	110
	¾ oz box	255	83
Lucky Charms	1 oz or about 1 c	201	110
Total	1 oz or about 1 c	352	100
Trix	1 oz or about 1 c	181	109
Wheaties	1 oz or about 1 c	354	99

Health Valley
COLD CEREAL

	Portion	Sodium (mg)	Calories
Amaranth Crunch w/raisins	1 oz or about ¼ c	10	120
amaranth flakes	1 oz or about ½ c	5	110
amaranth w/banana	1 oz or about ¼ c	5	114
bran			
w/apples & cinnamon	1 oz or about ¼ c	10	110
w/raisins	1 oz or about ¼ c	5	108
Fiber 7 Flakes	1 oz or about ½ c	10	113
Fruit Lites			
corn	½ oz or about ½ c	2	48
rice	½ oz or about ½ c	2	48
wheat	½ oz or about ½ c	2	48
granola *See* Real Granola, *below*			
Healthy Crunch			
w/almonds & dates	1 oz or about ¼ c	10	120
w/apples & cinnamon	1 oz or about ¼ c	10	120
oat bran flakes			
plain	1 oz or about ½ c	5	117
w/almonds & dates	1 oz or about ½ c	10	105
w/raisins	1 oz or about ½ c	10	105

	Portion	Sodium (mg)	Calories
Orangeola			
w/almonds & dates	1 oz or about ¼ c	10	120
w/banana & Hawaiian fruit	1 oz or about ¼ c	10	128
raisin bran flakes	1 oz or about ½ c	1	108
Real Granola			
w/almond crunch or w/Hawaiian fruit	1 oz or about ¼ c	5	123
w/raisins & nuts	1 oz or about ¼ c	5	120
Sprouts 7			
w/bananas & Hawaiian fruit	1 oz or about ¼ c	5	90
w/raisins	1 oz or about ¼ c	5	105
stoned-wheat flakes	1 oz or about ½ c	1	108
Swiss Breakfast			
raisin nut	1 oz or about ¼ c	10	120
tropical fruit	1 oz or about ¼ c	10	120
wheat bran/Millers Flakes	1 oz or about ½ c	15	118
wheat germ w/fiber, almonds & dates	1 oz or about ¼ c	15	92
wheat germ w/fiber, bananas & tropical fruit	1 oz or about ¼ c	15	100
HOT CEREAL			
hot oat bran w/apples	1 oz or about ¼ c	10	100
Heartland Cold Cereal			
Natural Cereal			
plain	1 oz or about ¼ c	72	123
	1 c	294	499
w/coconut	1 oz or about ¼ c	57	125
	1 c	213	463
w/raisins	1 oz or about ¼ c	58	120
	1 c	225	467

	Portion	Sodium (mg)	Calories
Kellogg's Cold Cereal			
All-Bran	1 oz or about ⅓ c	260	70
w/extra fiber	1 oz or about ½ c	270	60
w/fruit & almonds	1.3 oz or about ⅔ c	260	100
Apple Jacks	1 oz or about 1 c	125	110
Bran Buds	1 oz or about ⅓ c	170	70
bran flakes	1 oz or about ⅔ c	220	90
Cocoa Krispies	1 oz or about ¾ c	190	110
Corn Flakes			
regular	1 oz or about 1 c	290	110
honey & nut	1 oz or about ⅔ c	200	110
Corn Pops	1 oz or about 1 c	90	110
Cracklin' Oat Bran	1 oz or about ½ c	140	110
Crispix	1 oz or about 1 c	220	110
Froot Loops	1 oz or about 1 c	125	110
Frosted Flakes	1 oz or about ¾ c	200	110
Frosted Krispies	1 oz or about ¾ c	220	110
Frosted Mini-Wheats	1 oz = about 4 biscuits	5	100
Fruitful Bran	1.3 oz or about ⅔ c	230	110
Honey Smacks	1 oz or about ¾ c	70	110
Just Right			
Fruit, Nut, & Flake	1.3 oz or about ¾ c	190	140
Nugget & Flake	1 oz or about ⅔ c	190	100
Müeslix			
bran	1 oz or about ½ c	100	130
Five Grain	1 oz or about ½ c	60	150
Nutri-Grain			
almond raisin	1.4 oz or about ⅔ c	220	140

	Portion	Sodium (mg)	Calories
Nutri-Grain *(cont.)*			
corn	1 oz or about ½ c	170	100
wheat	1 oz or about ⅔ c	170	100
wheat & raisins	1.4 oz or about ⅔ c	170	130
Product 19	1 oz or about 1 c	320	100
raisin bran	1.4 oz or about ¾ c	220	120
Rice Krispies	1 oz or about 1 c	290	110
Special K	1 oz or about 1 c	230	110
Malt-O-Meal Hot Cereal			
Malt-O-Meal, plain or chocolate			
dry	1 T	1	38
cooked	1 c	2	122
	¾ c	2	92
Maltex			
Maltex hot cereal	1 oz	0	105
Maypo			
30-Second Oatmeal	1 oz	0	100
Vermont-Style Hot Oat Cereal	1 oz	0	105
Nabisco			
COLD CEREAL			
Fruit Wheats			
apple or strawberry	1 oz	15	100
raisin	1 oz	5	100
100% Bran	1 oz or about ½ c	190	70
Shredded Wheat 'n Bran	1 oz	0	110
Team	1 oz or about 1 c	190	110
Toasted Wheat & Raisins	1 oz	0	100
HOT CEREAL			
Cream of Rice	1 oz dry	0	100
Cream of Wheat			
regular	1 oz dry	130	100
instant	1 oz dry	0	100
Mix 'n Eat			
Original	1 oz dry	180	100
w/apple & cinnamon	1¼ oz dry	240	130
w/peach or w/strawberry	1¼ oz dry	200	140
w/brown sugar cinnamon	1¼ oz dry	180	130
w/maple brown sugar	1¼ oz dry	130	180

	Portion	Sodium (mg)	Calories
quick			
regular	1 oz dry	130	100
w/apples, raisins, & spice or w/maple brown sugar, artificially flavored	1 oz dry	0	110
Nature Valley Cold Cereal			
granola, toasted oat mixture	1 oz or about ⅓ c	58	126
	1 c	232	503
Post Cold Cereal			
Alpha-Bits	1 oz	180	110
C.W. Post Hearty Granola			
plain	1 oz	80	130
w/raisins	1 oz	80	120
Cocoa Pebbles	1 oz	160	110
Fruit & Fibre: dates, raisins, walnuts; Harvest Medley; Mountain Trail; or tropical fruit	1 oz	180	90
Fruity Pebbles	1 oz	150	110
granola See C.W. Post Hearty Granola, above			
Grape-Nuts			
regular	1 oz	190	110
raisin	1 oz	140	100
Grape-Nuts Flakes	1 oz	160	100
Honeycomb	1 oz	160	110
Natural Bran Flakes	1 oz	230	90
Natural Raisin Bran	1 oz	180	80
oat flakes, fortified	1 oz	250	110
Post Toasties	1 oz	280	110
Super Golden Crisp	1 oz or about ⅞ c	45	110
Quaker Oats			
COLD CEREAL			
100% Natural Cereal			
plain	1 oz or about ¼ c	43	127
w/apples & cinnamon	1 oz or about ¼ c	13	126
w/raisins & dates	1 oz or about ¼ c	14	123
bran, unprocessed	.25 oz	0	8
Cap'n Crunch			
regular	1 oz or about ¾ c	241	113
peanut butter	1 oz or about ¾ c	281	119
w/Crunchberries	1 oz or about ¾ c	247	113
Crunchy Bran	1 oz or about ¾ c	316	89

	Portion	Sodium (mg)	Calories
Life, plain or cinnamon	1 oz or about ⅔ c	186	101
Oat Squares	1 oz	159	105
HOT CEREAL			
oat bran	1 oz	1	92
oatmeal, instant, prepared			
regular	1 oz	270	94
w/apples & cinnamon	1.25 oz	128	118
w/artificial maple & brown sugar	1.5 oz	320	152
w/peaches & cream	1 oz	179	129
w/raisins & spice	1 oz	266	149
w/raisins, dates, & walnuts	1 oz	216	141
w/strawberries & cream	1 oz	204	129
Quaker Oats, Quick & Old Fashioned	1 oz	1	99
Whole Wheat Hot Natural	⅓ c dry or ⅔ c cooked	1	92
Ralston Purina *COLD CEREAL*			
Bran Chex	1 oz or about ⅔ c	263	91
	1 c	455	156
Cookie-Crisp	1 oz or about 1 c	195	114
Corn Chex	1 oz or about 1 c	271	111
	¾ oz box	204	84
cornflakes	1 oz or about 1 c	271	111
40% bran flakes	1 oz or about ¾ c	264	92
	1 c	456	159
raisin bran	1⅓ oz or about ¾ c	328	120
	1 c	486	178
Rice Chex	1 oz or about 1⅛ c	237	112
	⅞ oz box	207	98
sugar-frosted flakes	1 oz or about ¾ c	184	111
	1 c	247	149
Tasteeos	1 oz or about 1¼ c	216	111
	1 c	183	94
Waffelos	1 oz or about 1 c	118	115
Wheat Chex	1 oz or about ⅔ c	190	104
	1 c	308	169

	Portion	Sodium (mg)	Calories
Wheat 'n Raisin Chex	1⅓ oz or about ¾ c	214	130
	1 c	306	185
HOT CEREAL			
Ralston			
dry	¼ c	3	102
cooked	1 c	4	134
	¾ c	3	100
Roman Meal Hot Cereal			
Roman Meal			
plain			
dry	⅓ c	2	100
cooked	1 c	3	147
	¾ c	2	111
w/oats			
dry	¼ c	5	85
cooked	1 c	10	169
	¾ c	7	127
Sun Country Granola			
w/almonds	1 oz	11	130
w/raisins	1 oz	10	125
w/raisins & dates	1 oz	9	123
Sunshine			
shredded wheat			
regular	1 biscuit	0	90
bite size	⅔ c	0	110
U.S. Mills			
See also Erewhon, *above*			
Skinner's raisin bran			
regular	1 oz or about ½ c	45	110
no salt added	1 oz or about ½ c	2	100
Uncle Sam cereal	1 oz or about ½ c	65	110
Wheatena Hot Cereal			
Wheatena			
dry	¼ c	4	125
cooked	1 oz	0	100

◻ BREAKFAST FOODS, PREPARED
See also EGGS & EGG SUBSTITUTES; FAST FOODS

	Portion	Sodium (mg)	Calories
French toast, homemade	1 slice	257	155
pancakes			
from mix			
plain	1 (7 T batter)	431	159
buckwheat	1 (4″ diam)	125	55
extra light	3 (4″ diam)	698	190
homemade, plain	1 (4″ diam)	115	60
waffles			
from mix	1 (7″ diam)	515	205
frozen	1	235	95
homemade	1 (7″ diam)	445	245

■ BRAND NAME

Arrowhead Mills Pancake Mixes

	Portion	Sodium (mg)	Calories
buckwheat	½ c	500	270
Griddle Lite	½ c	417	260
multigrain	½ c	830	350
triticale	½ c	495	270

Aunt Jemima
FRENCH TOAST, FROZEN

	Portion	Sodium (mg)	Calories
original flavor	3 oz	554	166
cinnamon swirl	3 oz	516	171
raisin	3 oz	492	172

PANCAKE & WAFFLE MIXES

	Portion	Sodium (mg)	Calories
original flavor	1.3 oz	609	116
buckwheat	1.3 oz	773	143
buttermilk	1.3 oz	698	122
whole-wheat	1.3 oz	892	161

PANCAKE BATTER, FROZEN

	Portion	Sodium (mg)	Calories
original flavor	3.6 oz	763	183
blueberry	3.6 oz	688	204
buttermilk	3.6 oz	778	180

PANCAKES, FROZEN

	Portion	Sodium (mg)	Calories
original flavor	3.48 oz	801	211
blueberry	3.48 oz	826	220

WAFFLES, FROZEN

	Portion	Sodium (mg)	Calories
original flavor	2	591	173
apple & cinnamon	2	616	176
blueberry	2	684	175
buttermilk	2	615	179

Fearn Pancake Mixes

	Portion	Sodium (mg)	Calories
buckwheat	½ c dry	740	235
Rich Earth	½ c dry	615	190
stone-ground whole-wheat	½ c dry	740	220

	Portion	Sodium (mg)	Calories
unbleached wheat & soya	½ c dry	740	235
Featherweight			
pancake mix	3 (4″ diam)	70	130
Health Valley			
7 Sprouted Grains buttermilk pancake & biscuit mix	1 oz	170	100
Kellogg's			
EGGO FROZEN WAFFLES			
apple cinnamon	1	300	130
buttermilk	1	300	120
Homestyle	1	300	120

POP-TARTS See DESSERTS: CAKES, PASTRIES, & PIES

Nabisco Toastettes *See* DESSERTS: CAKES, PASTRIES, & PIES

Swanson
GREAT STARTS BREAKFAST SANDWICHES

egg, Canadian bacon, & cheese/muffin	4.1 oz	780	300
sausage, egg, & cheese/biscuit	5½ oz	1,400	460
steak, egg, & cheese/muffin	4.9 oz	770	380

GREAT STARTS BREAKFASTS

French toast (cinnamon swirl)	6½ oz	660	470
French toast w/sausages	6½ oz	640	450
omelets w/cheese sauce & ham	7 oz	1,200	380
pancakes & blueberry sauce	7 oz	800	410
pancakes & sausages	6 oz	900	470
scrambled eggs & sausage w/hashed brown potatoes	6¼ oz	780	430
Spanish-style omelet	7¾ oz	800	240

❑ BROWNIES *See* COOKIES, BARS, & BROWNIES

❑ BUTTER & MARGARINE SPREADS

Butter
See also NUTS & NUT-BASED BUTTERS, FLOURS, MEALS, MILKS, PASTES, & POWDERS; SEEDS & SEED-BASED BUTTERS, FLOURS, & MEALS

salted or unsalted	1 stick = 4 oz or about ½ c	937	813
	1 t	41	36

	Portion	Sodium (mg)	Calories
whipped, salted	1 stick = 4 oz or about ½ c	625	542
	1 t	31	27

Margarine

IMITATION (ABOUT 40% FAT)

all kinds	1 c	2,226	801
	1 t	46	17

REGULAR
Hard, Stick or Brick

coconut, safflower, coconut (hydrogenated), & palm (hydrogenated)	1 stick	1,070	815
	1 t	44	34
corn (hydrogenated)	1 stick	1,070	815
	1 t	44	34
corn & corn (hydrogenated)	1 t	44	34
	1 stick	1,070	815
corn, soybean (hydrogenated), & cottonseed (hydrogenated)			
salted	1 stick	1,070	815
	1 t	44	34
unsalted	1 stick	2	810
	1 t	tr	34
lard (hydrogenated)	1 stick	1,070	831
	1 t	44	35
safflower & soybean (hydrogenated)	1 stick	1,070	815
	1 t	44	34
safflower, soybean (hydrogenated), & cottonseed (hydrogenated)	1 stick	1,070	815
	1 t	44	34
safflower, soybean, soybean (hydrogenated), & cottonseed (hydrogenated)	1 stick	1,070	815
	1 t	44	34
soybean (hydrogenated)	1 stick	1,070	815
	1 t	44	34
soybean (hydrogenated) & cottonseed	1 stick	1,070	815
	1 t	44	34
soybean (hydrogenated) & cottonseed (hydrogenated)	1 stick	1,070	815
	1 t	44	34
soybean (hydrogenated) & palm (hydrogenated)	1 stick	1,070	815
	1 t	44	34

	Portion	Sodium (mg)	Calories
soybean & soybean (hydrogenated)	1 stick t 1	1,070 44	815 34
soybean (hydrogenated), corn, & cottonseed (hydrogenated)	1 stick 1 t	1,070 44	815 34
soybean (hydrogenated), cottonseed (hydrogenated), & soybean	1 stick 1 t	1,070 44	815 34
soybean (hydrogenated), palm (hydrogenated), & palm	1 stick 1 t	1,070 44	815 34
sunflower, soybean (hydrogenated), & cottonseed (hydrogenated)	1 stick 1 t	1,070 44	815 34
Liquid, Bottle			
soybean (hydrogenated), soybean, & cottonseed	1 c 1 t	1,773 37	1,637 34
Soft, Tub			
corn & corn (hydrogenated)	1 c 1 t	2,449 51	1,626 34
safflower & safflower (hydrogenated)	1 c 1 t	2,449 51	1,626 34
safflower, cottonseed (hydrogenated), & peanut (hydrogenated)	1 c 1 t	2,449 51	1,626 34
soybean (hydrogenated)			
salted	1 c 1 t	2,449 51	1,626 34
unsalted	1 c 1 t	63 1	1,626 34
soybean (hydrogenated) & cottonseed	1 c 1 t	2,449 51	1,626 34
soybean (hydrogenated) & cottonseed (hydrogenated)			
salted	1 c 1 t	2,449 51	1,626 34
unsalted	1 c 1 t	63 1	1,626 34
soybean (hydrogenated) & safflower	1 c 1 t	2,449 51	1,626 34

	Portion	Sodium (mg)	Calories
soybean (hydrogenated), cottonseed (hydrogenated), & soybean	1 c 1 t	2,449 51	1,626 34
soybean (hydrogenated), palm (hydrogenated), & palm	1 c 1 t	2,449 51	1,626 34
soybean, soybean (hydrogenated), & cottonseed (hydrogenated)	1 c 1 t	2,449 51	1,626 34
sunflower, cottonseed (hydrogenated), & peanut (hydrogenated)	1 c 1 t	2,449 51	1,626 34

SPREAD, MARGARINELIKE (ABOUT 60% FAT)

	Portion	Sodium (mg)	Calories
all kinds, stick or tub	1 c 1 t	2,276 48	1,236 26

▪ BRAND NAME

Blue Bonnet Margarine
Butter Blend, soft or stick

	Portion	Sodium (mg)	Calories
salted	1 T	95	90
unsalted	1 T	10	90
margarine			
regular, soft or stick	1 T	95	100
diet	1 T	100	50
whipped, soft or stick	1 T	70	70
spread			
52% fat	1 T	110	80
Light Tasty, 52% vegetable oil	1 T	100	60
stick, 75% fat	1 T	95	90
stick, 70% fat	1 T	95	90
whipped, 60% fat	1 T	55	50

Fleischmann's Margarine
regular, salted

	Portion	Sodium (mg)	Calories
squeeze	1 T	85	100
stick or soft	1 T	95	100
regular, unsalted: stick, soft, or squeeze	1 T	0	100
diet	1 T	100	50
diet w/lite salt	1 T	50	50
whipped, salted	1 T	60	70
whipped, unsalted	1 T	0	70

	Portion	Sodium (mg)	Calories
Land O'Lakes			
butter			
regular, salted	1 T	115	100
regular, unsalted	1 T	2	100
whipped, salted	1 T	75	60
whipped, unsalted	1 T	1	60
Country Morning Blend margarine			
soft, tub, salted	1 T	85	90
soft, tub, unsalted	1 T	1	90
stick, salted	1 T	115	100
stick, unsalted	1 T	1	100
Mazola Margarine			
regular, salted	1 T	100	100
regular, unsalted	1 T	0	100
diet	1 T	130	50

❑ **CAKES** *See* **DESSERTS: CAKES, PASTRIES, & PIES**

❑ **CANDIED FRUIT** *See* **BAKING INGREDIENTS**

❑ **CANDY**

	Portion	Sodium (mg)	Calories
butterscotch	6 pieces	19	116
butterscotch chips	1 oz	20	150
caramels			
plain or chocolate	3	63	112
plain or chocolate w/nuts	2	57	120
chocolate			
chocolate fudge center	1	68	129
chocolate fudge w/nuts center	1	57	127
coconut center	1	55	123
cream center	1	2	102
fondant center	1	52	115
vanilla cream center	1	48	114
chocolate chips			
chocolate-flavored	¼ c	10	195
dark	1 oz	64	148
milk chocolate	¼ c	55	218
semisweet	1 c or 6 oz (60 chips/oz)	24	860
chocolate kisses	6	25	154

	Portion	Sodium (mg)	Calories
chocolate stars	7	26	145
chocolate-covered almonds	1 oz	17	159
chocolate-covered Brazil nuts	1 oz	13	162
English toffee	1 oz	79	193
fondant, uncoated (mints, candy corn, other)	1 oz	57	105
fudge			
chocolate, plain	1 oz	54	115
chocolate w/nuts	1 oz	48	119
vanilla	1 oz	58	111
vanilla w/nuts	1 oz	52	119
granola bars See COOKIES, BARS, & BROWNIES			
gum drops	1 oz	10	100
hard candy	1 oz	7	110
	6 pieces	9	108
jelly beans	1 oz	7	105
	10	3	66
malted milk balls	14	28	135
marshmallows	1 oz	25	90
	1 large	4	25
mints	14	47	104
peanut brittle	1 oz	9	123
sugar-coated almonds	7	6	128

▪ BRAND NAME

NOTE: Candies may be listed under product name (e.g., Kit Kat) or company name (e.g., Hershey).

	Portion	Sodium (mg)	Calories
Almond Joy	1 oz	58	136
Baby Ruth	½ bar	60	130
Baker's chocolate See BAKING INGREDIENTS			
Beech-Nut			
cough drops, all flavors	1	0	10
gum, all flavors	1 piece	0	10
Beechies candy-coated gum, all flavors	1 piece	0	6
Bonkers!, all flavors	1 piece	0	20
Breath Savers Mints, sugar-free, all flavors	1	0	8
Bubble Yum bubble gum, all flavors			
regular	1 piece	0	25
sugarless	1 piece	0	20
Butterfinger	½ bar	60	130
Care-Free			
sugarless bubble gum, all flavors	1 piece	0	10
sugarless gum, all flavors	1 piece	0	8
Charleston Chew!	½ piece	40	120

	Portion	Sodium (mg)	Calories
Hershey			
chocolate chips & unsweetened chocolate *See* baking ingredients			
chocolate Kisses	9 or 1.5 oz	33	222
Krackel	1.65 oz	73	249
milk chocolate	1.65 oz	35	254
milk chocolate w/almonds	1.55 oz	55	246
Special Dark sweet chocolate	1.45 oz	4	221
Junior Mints	12	10	120
Kit Kat	1.13 oz	28	162
	1.6 oz	53	244
Life Savers			
lollipops, all flavors	1	10	45
milk chocolate stars	13	35	160
roll candy, all flavors, regular or sugar-free	1 piece	0–10	8
Mounds	1 oz	53	135
Mr. Goodbar	1.27 oz	16	198
	1.85 oz	18	296
big block	2 oz	25	300
Nestlé			
Crunch	1.06 oz	50	160
milk chocolate	1.07 oz	25	160
milk chocolate w/almonds	1 oz	20	150
Pearson's			
Carmel Nip	4	70	120
Chocolate Parfait	4	70	120
Coffee Nip	4	70	120
Licorice Nip	4	70	120
Planters			
Old Fashioned peanut candy	1 oz	70	140
peanut bar			
regular	1.6 oz	70	230
honey roasted	1.6 oz	145	230
Sweet 'n Crunchy	1.6 oz	110	250
Pom Poms	½ box	70	100
Reese's			
Peanut Butter Cup	1.8 oz	148	281
peanut butter–flavored chips	¼ c	108	228
Pieces	1.95 oz	83	270
Rolo	9 pieces or 1.93 oz	94	264
Skor	1.4 oz	92	220
Sugar Babies	1 pkg	85	180
Sugar Daddy	1	85	150
Thousand Dollar	1½ oz	75	200
Whatchamacallit	1.8 oz	122	270

	Portion	Sodium (mg)	Calories

❑ **CANNED MEATS** *See* PROCESSED MEAT & POULTRY PRODUCTS

❑ **CEREAL, BREAKFAST** *See* BREAKFAST CEREALS, COLD & HOT

❑ **CHEESE & CHEESE FOODS**

Natural Cheese

	Portion	Sodium (mg)	Calories
bleu	1 oz	396	100
	1 c, crumbled, not packed	1,884	477
brick	1″ cube	96	64
	1 oz	159	105
Brie	1 oz	178	95
	4½ oz	806	427
Camembert	1 oz	239	85
	3⅓ oz	320	114
caraway	1 oz	196	107
cheddar	1 oz	176	114
	1 c, shredded, not packed	701	455
Cheshire	1 oz	198	110
Colby	1″ cube	104	68
	1 oz	171	112
cottage			
creamed, small curd	4 oz	457	117
	1 c, not packed	850	217
fruit added	4 oz	457	140
	1 c, not packed	915	279
dry curd	4 oz	14	96
	1 c, not packed	19	123
low-fat			
2%	4 oz	459	101
	1 c, not packed	918	203
1%	4 oz	459	82
	1 c, not packed	918	164
cream	1 oz	84	99
	3 oz	251	297
Edam	1 oz	274	101
	7 oz	1,911	706
feta, from sheep's milk	1 oz	316	75

	Portion	Sodium (mg)	Calories
gjetost, from goats' & cows' milk	1 oz	170	132
	8 oz	1,362	1,057
Gouda	1 oz	232	101
	7 oz	1,622	705
Gruyère	1 oz	95	117
	6 oz	571	702
Limburger	1 oz	227	93
	8 oz	1,816	742
Monterey Jack	1 oz	152	106
	6 oz	912	635
mozzarella	1 oz	106	80
low-moisture	1″ cube	73	56
	1 oz	118	90
part skim	1″ cube	93	49
	1 oz	150	79
part skim	1 oz	132	72
Muenster	1 oz	178	104
	6 oz	1,067	626
Neufchâtel	1 oz	113	74
	3 oz	339	221
Parmesan			
grated	1 T	93	23
	1 oz	528	129
hard	1 oz	454	111
	5 oz	2,274	557
Port du Salut	1 oz	151	100
	6 oz	908	598
provolone	1 oz	248	100
	6 oz	1,488	598
ricotta			
whole milk	½ c	307	216
part skim milk	½ c	155	171
Romano, hard	1 oz	340	110
	5 oz	1,704	549
Roquefort, from sheep's milk	1 oz	513	105
	3 oz	1,538	314
Swiss	1″ cube	39	56
	1 oz	74	107
Tilsit	1 oz	213	96
	6 oz	1,280	578

whey *See* MILK, MILK SUBSTITUTES, & MILK PRODUCTS

Process Cheese & Cheese Food

CHEESE FOOD

American			
cold pack	1 oz	274	94
	8 oz	2,193	752
pasteurized process	1 oz	337	93
	8 oz	2,700	745

	Portion	Sodium (mg)	Calories
Swiss, pasteurized process	1 oz	440	92
	8 oz	3,523	734
CHEESE SPREAD			
American, pasteurized process	1 oz	381	82
	5 oz	1,910	412
PASTEURIZED PROCESS CHEESE			
American	1" cube	250	66
	1 oz	406	106
pimiento	1" cube	250	66
	1 oz	405	106
Swiss	1" cube	245	60
	1 oz	388	95

▪ BRAND NAME

Armour
cheddar

	Portion	Sodium (mg)	Calories
regular	1 oz	180	110
lower salt	1 oz	106	110
Colby			
regular	1 oz	170	110
lower salt	1 oz	120	110
Monterey Jack			
regular	1 oz	160	110
lower salt	1 oz	111	110

Bonbel *See* Fromageries Bel, *below*
Featherweight

	Portion	Sodium (mg)	Calories
cheddar, low-sodium	1 oz	5	110

Friendship
cottage cheese

	Portion	Sodium (mg)	Calories
California style, 4% milk fat	½ c	390	120
Friendship 'n Fruit	6 oz	430	100
low-fat			
regular or lactose-reduced, both 1% milk fat	½ c	360	90
large curd pot style, 2% milk fat	½ c	440	100
w/pineapple, 4% milk fat	½ c	270	140
cream cheese	1 oz	70	103
farmer cheese	½ c	356	160
natural hoop cheese, ½% milk fat	4 oz	10	84

Fromageries Bel

	Portion	Sodium (mg)	Calories
Babybel	1 oz	227	91
Bombino	1 oz	227	103
Bonbel	1 oz	227	100

	Portion	Sodium (mg)	Calories
cheddar	1 oz	227	110
Edam	1 oz	227	100
Gouda	1 oz	227	110
Mini Babybel	¾ oz	170	74
Mini Bonbel	¾ oz	170	74
Mini Gouda	¾ oz	170	80
Reduced Mini	¾ oz	170	45
Land O'Lakes			
NATURAL CHEESE			
brick	1 oz	160	110
cheddar	1 oz	175	110
Colby	1 oz	170	110
Edam	1 oz	275	100
Gouda	1 oz	230	100
Monterey Jack	1 oz	150	110
mozzarella, low-moisture, part skim	1 oz	150	80
Muenster	1 oz	180	100
provolone	1 oz	250	100
Swiss	1 oz	75	110
PROCESS CHEESE & CHEESE FOOD			
American	1 oz	405	110
American Swiss	1 oz	445	100
Golden Velvet cheese spread	1 oz	380	80
Jalapeño cheese food	1 oz	360	90
La Chedda cheese food	1 oz	90	360
onion cheese food	1 oz	330	90
pepperoni cheese food	1 oz	395	90
salami cheese food	1 oz	100	400
Wispride Cold Pack Cheese Food			
sharp cheddar	1 oz	210	100

❑ **CHICKEN** *See* POULTRY, FRESH
& PROCESSED

❑ **CHUTNEYS** *See* PICKLES, OLIVES,
RELISHES, & CHUTNEYS

❑ **COATINGS, SEASONED**
See BREADCRUMBS, CROUTONS,
STUFFINGS, & SEASONED COATINGS

	Portion	Sodium (mg)	Calories

❑ **CONDIMENTS** *See* SAUCES, GRAVIES, & CONDIMENTS

❑ **COOKIES, BARS, & BROWNIES**

	Portion	Sodium (mg)	Calories
animal cookies	15	113	120
arrowroot cookies	2	24	47
brownies			
butterscotch	1 oz	98	115
chocolate, from mix	1.1 oz	95	130
chocolate, w/nuts			
commercial, frosted	0.9 oz	59	100
homemade, w/vegetable oil	0.7 oz	51	95
chocolate chip cookies			
commercial	4 (2¼″ diam)	140	180
from refrigerator dough	4 (2¼″ diam)	173	225
homemade, w/vegetable shortening	4 (2⅓″ diam)	82	185
chocolate cookies	1	29	93
chocolate sandwich cookies	1	63	49
coconut bars	1	33	109
fig bars	1	45	53
	4 = 2 oz	180	210
gingersnaps			
commercial	2	80	59
homemade	1	20	34
graham crackers	2	66	60
chocolate-covered	1	53	62
granola bars	1	67	109
macaroons	1	7	90
molasses cookies	1	125	137
oatmeal chocolate chip cookies	1	23	57
oatmeal cookies			
commercial	1	69	80
from mix	2	45	130
homemade	1	37	62
oatmeal raisin cookies			
from refrigerator dough	1	37	61
homemade	4 (2⅝″ diam)	148	245
peanut butter bars	1	116	198
peanut butter cookies			
from refrigerator dough	1	57	50
homemade	4 = 1.7 oz	142	245
peanut cookies	1	21	57
sandwich-type cookies, chocolate or vanilla	4 = 1.4 oz	189	195
shortbread cookies			
commercial	4 small	123	155
homemade, w/margarine	2 large	125	145

	Portion	Sodium (mg)	Calories
social tea cookies	2	33	43
sugar cookies			
from mix	2	75	120
from refrigerator dough	4 = 1.7 oz	261	235
homemade	1	64	89
sugar wafers	2	36	92
vanilla cream sandwich cookies	1	68	69
vanilla wafers	5	50	92
Vienna dream bars, from mix	1	65	90

▪ BRAND NAME

Famous Amos

	Portion	Sodium (mg)	Calories
chocolate chip w/macadamia nuts	1 oz	70	152
chocolate chip w/pecans	1 oz	57	151
chocolate chip, no nuts, extra chips	1 oz	79	147
oatmeal w/cinnamon & raisins	1 oz	82	133

Health Valley

	Portion	Sodium (mg)	Calories
fruit bars			
apple	2	35	165
date	2	40	180
raisin	2	35	160
Fruit Jumbos			
almonds & dates	1	30	75
oat bran	1	35	70
raisins & nuts	1	35	75
tropical fruit	1	26	80
graham crackers			
amaranth	7	110	110
oat bran	7	85	120
Jumbos			
amaranth	1	30	83
cinnamon	1	35	70
peanut butter	1	35	70
tofu cookies	4	80	145
wheat-free cookies	4	80	180

Hershey New Trail Granola Snack Bars

	Portion	Sodium (mg)	Calories
chocolate-covered chocolate chip	1	60	200
chocolate-covered cocoa creme	1	70	190
chocolate-covered cookies & cream	1	85	200
chocolate-covered peanut butter	1	90	200

	Portion	Sodium (mg)	Calories
Kellogg's Rice Krispies Bars			
chocolate chip	1	110	120
Cocoa Krispies chocolate chip	1	110	120
peanut butter	1	115	130
Nabisco			
Almost Home Family-Style cookies			
fudge & nut brownies	1	75	160
fudge & vanilla creme sandwiches	1	110	140
fudge chocolate chip cookies	2	130	130
iced Dutch apple fruit sticks	1	40	70
oatmeal raisin cookies	2	100	130
Old Fashioned sugar cookies	2	150	130
peanut butter chocolate chip cookies	2	100	140
Real chocolate chip cookies	2	100	130
Apple Newtons	1	45	110
Barnum's Animals (animal crackers)	11	120	130
Bugs Bunny graham cookies	9	130	120
Cameo creme sandwiches	2	80	140
Chewy Chips Ahoy!	2	110	130
Chips 'n More	2	70	150
chocolate grahams	3	70	150
chocolate snaps	7	100	130
Cinnamon Treats	2	80	60
Cookies 'n Fudge	3	80	150
devil's food cakes	1	70	110
Famous chocolate wafers	5	200	130
Giggles vanilla sandwich cookies	2	50	140
graham crackers	2	115	60
Honey Maid graham crackers	2	90	60
I Screams n' You Screams Double Dip chocolate creme sandwiches	2	70	150
Lorna Doone shortbread	4	130	140
Mallomars	2	35	130
National arrowroot biscuits	6	80	130
Old Fashion ginger snaps	4	200	120
Oreo chocolate sandwich cookies	3	170	140
Oreo mint creme chocolate sandwich cookies	2	160	150
Pantry molasses cookies	2	130	130
pecan shortbread cookies	2	80	150
Pinwheels	1	35	130
Social Tea biscuits	6	105	130

	Portion	Sodium (mg)	Calories
Pepperidge Farm			
ASSORTMENT COOKIES			
Champagne	2	60	95
Original Pirouettes	2	60	110
Seville	2	50	100
DISTINCTIVE COOKIES			
Bordeaux	3	70	110
Brussels	3	100	160
Chessmen	3	80	130
Geneva	3	80	190
Lido	2	90	190
Milano	3	80	180
Nassau	2	90	170
Orleans	3	30	90
FRUIT COOKIES			
apricot-raspberry	3	80	150
KITCHEN HEARTH COOKIES			
date pecan	3	180	160
raisin bran	3	80	160
OLD FASHIONED COOKIES			
brownie chocolate nut	3	70	160
chocolate chip	3	90	150
chocolate chocolate chip	3	80	160
Gingerman	3	80	100
hazelnut	3	110	170
Irish oatmeal	3	120	140
Lemon Nut Crunch	3	80	170
Molasses Crisps	3	80	100
oatmeal raisin	3	170	170
shortbread	3	90	150
sugar	3	120	150
SPECIAL COLLECTION COOKIES			
Almond Supreme	2	50	140
Chocolate Chunk Pecan	2	50	130
milk chocolate macadamia	2	80	140
Pillsbury			
chocolate chip cookies	3	105	210
fudge brownies	1	115	140
oatmeal raisin cookies	3	180	210
peanut butter cookies	3	210	210
sugar cookies	3	210	210

	Portion	Sodium (mg)	Calories
Quaker Oats			
CHEWY GRANOLA BARS			
chocolate chip	1	90	128
chocolate, graham, & marsh-mallow	1	108	126
chunky nut & raisin	1	86	131
honey & oats	1	95	125
peanut butter	1	116	128
raisin & cinnamon	1	92	128
GRANOLA DIPPS BARS			
caramel nut	1	81	148
chocolate chip	1	78	139
peanut butter	1	74	170
peanut butter & chocolate chip	1	102	174
Sunshine			
animal crackers	14	180	120
butter-flavored cookies	4	150	120
Chip-A-Roos	2	100	130
cinnamon graham crackers	4, after breaking	95	70
Country Style oatmeal cookies	2	125	110
fig bars	2	60	90
ginger snaps	5	120	100
Golden Fruit raisin biscuits	2, after breaking	80	150
honey graham crackers	4, after breaking	90	60
Hydrox	3	140	160
Mallopuffs	2	100	140
sugar wafers	3	40	130
vanilla wafers	6	105	130
Vienna fingers	2	125	140

❏ **CORNMEAL** *See* FLOURS & CORNMEALS

❏ **CRACKERS**

	Portion	Sodium (mg)	Calories
bread sticks *See* BREADS, ROLLS, BISCUITS, & MUFFINS			
cheese, plain	10 (1″ square)	112	50
cheese & peanut butter sandwich	1	90	40
graham *See* COOKIES, BARS, & BROWNIES			
matzo	1	tr	117

	Portion	Sodium (mg)	Calories
melba toast, plain	1	44	20
oyster	10	83	33
rice wafers	3	8	31
rusk	1	22	38
rye crisp	¼ large square	112	40
rye wafers, whole-grain	2 = ½ oz	115	55
saltines	4	165	50
snack-type crackers, standard, round	1	30	15
soda, unsalted tops	10	208	120
taco shells *See* BREADS, ROLLS, BISCUITS, & MUFFINS			
tortillas *See* BREADS, ROLLS, BISCUITS, & MUFFINS			
wheat, thin	4	69	35
whole-wheat wafers	2	59	35
zwieback *See* INFANT & TODDLER FOODS			

▪ BRAND NAME

Cracottes

regular	1	20	12
salt-free	1	<1	12
whole-wheat	1	21	13

Featherweight

bran wafers	4	2	50
crackers	2	1	30

Health Valley

Cheese Wheels	13	120	150
herb			
regular	13	160	135
no salt	13	30	135
honey graham	13	125	120
sesame			
regular	13	150	130
no salt	13	20	130
7-Grain Vegetable			
regular	13	125	130
no salt	13	20	125
stoned-wheat			
regular	13	85	135
no salt	13	10	135

Nabisco

Bacon-Flavored Thins	7	210	70
Better Blue Cheese	10	260	70
Better Cheddars	11	220	70
Better Cheddars 'n' Bacon	10	210	70

	Portion	Sodium (mg)	Calories
Better Nacho	9	220	70
Better Swiss Cheese	10	230	70
Cheese Peanut Butter Sandwich	2	150	70
Cheese Tid-Bits	16	200	70
Cheese Wheat Thins	9	220	70
Chicken in a Biskit	7	115	70
Crown Pilot	1	65	60
Dandy Soup & Oyster	20	220	60
Dip in a Chip Cheese 'n Chive	8	130	70
Escort	3	110	80
graham or Honey Maid graham crackers *See* COOKIES, BARS, & BROWNIES			
Great Crisps! *See* SNACKS			
Holland Rusk	1	35	60
Meal Mates	3	140	70
Nips *See* SNACKS			
Nutty Wheat Thins	7	250	80
Oysterettes	18	130	60
Premium saltines			
regular	5	180	60
low-salt	5	115	60
Ritz			
regular	4	120	70
cheese	5	120	70
low-salt	4	60	70
Royal Lunch Milk	1	80	60
Sea Rounds	1	140	60
Sociables	6	130	70
Toasted Peanut Butter Sandwich	2	150	70
Triscuits			
regular	3	90	60
low-salt	3	35	60
Twigs, sesame or cheese	5	200	70
Uneeda Biscuit, unsalted tops	3	100	60
Vegetable Thins	7	100	70
Waverly	4	160	70
Wheat Thins			
regular	8	120	70
low-salt	8	60	70
Wheatsworth	5	135	70
Pepperidge Farm			
butter-flavored thin crackers	4	100	80
English water biscuits	4	90	70
Hearty wheat crackers	4	180	100
sesame crackers	4	110	80
Snack Sticks *See* SNACKS			
three-cracker assortment	4	180	100
Tiny Goldfish *See* SNACKS			

	Portion	Sodium (mg)	Calories
Pillsbury			
bread sticks *See* BREADS, ROLLS, BISCUITS, & MUFFINS			
Quaker Oats			
rice cakes, lightly salted			
plain	1	36	35
multigrain	1	29	34
sesame	1	30	35
rice cakes, unsalted, plain	1	0	35
Sunshine			
American Heritage			
cheddar	5	150	80
sesame	4	125	70
Cheez-It	12	135	70
Hi Ho	4	125	80
Krispy saltines	5	210	60
oyster & soup	16	190	60
Wheats	8	190	80

❏ **CREAM & CREAM SUBSTITUTES**
See MILK, MILK SUBSTITUTES,
& MILK PRODUCTS

❏ **CROUTONS** *See* BREADCRUMBS,
CROUTONS, STUFFINGS, & SEASONED
COATINGS

❏ **CUSTARDS** *See* DESSERTS: CUSTARDS,
GELATINS, PUDDINGS, & PIE FILLINGS

❏ **DELI MEATS** *See* PROCESSED MEAT
& POULTRY PRODUCTS

❏ **DESSERTS: CAKES, PASTRIES,
& PIES**

Cake & Coffee Cake

	Portion	Sodium (mg)	Calories
angel food			
from mix	whole (9¾" diam tube)	3,226	1,510
	¹⁄₁₂ cake	269	125
homemade	2.1 oz	161	161

	Portion	Sodium (mg)	Calories
applesauce spice, from mix	1/12 cake	300	250
banana, from mix	1/12 cake	290	250
w/buttercream icing	1.8 oz	122	181
Boston cream pie	3.9 oz	205	332
butter brickle, from mix	1/12 cake	255	260
butter pecan, from mix	1/12 cake	250	250
caramel, from mix	1.6 oz	137	173
w/caramel icing	1.9 oz	139	208
carrot			
from mix	1/12 cake	253	187
homemade, w/cream cheese icing	whole (10" diam tube)	4,470	6,175
	1/16 cake	279	385
cheesecake			
commercial	whole (9" diam)	2,464	3,350
	1/12 cake	204	280
from mix	1/8 cake	366	300
cherry chip, from mix	1/12 cake	265	180
chocolate			
from mix	1/12 cake	450	250
w/icing, from mix	1.3 oz cupcake	121	129
chocolate chip, from mix	1/12 cake	249	189
chocolate fudge bundt ring, from mix	1/16 cake	315	270
chocolate fudge w/vanilla icing, from mix	1/6 cake	295	280
chocolate macaroon bundt ring, from mix	1/16 cake	315	250
chocolate mint, from mix	1/12 cake	370	250
chocolate pudding, from mix	1/6 cake	255	230
cinnamon streusel, from mix	1/8 cake	225	250
coffee cake, crumb, from mix	whole (15.1 oz)	1,853	1,385
	1/6 cake	310	230
cottage pudding, homemade	1/8 cake	161	186
w/chocolate sauce	1/8 cake & 1 T sauce	172	235
w/strawberry sauce	1/8 cake & 1 T sauce	163	204
devil's food, homemade	2.1 oz	160	227
devil's food, w/chocolate icing			
from mix, made w/margarine	whole, 2-layer (8" or 9" diam)	2,900	3,755
	1/16 cake	181	235
	1.2 oz cupcake	92	120
homemade	2.1 oz	108	233

	Portion	Sodium (mg)	Calories
fruitcake			
dark, homemade	3 lbs	2,123	5,185
	1½ oz	67	165
light	1.4 oz	77	156
German chocolate, from mix	1/12 cake	340	250
gingerbread			
from mix	whole (8" square)	1,733	1,575
	1/9 cake	192	175
homemade	2½ oz	99	267
lemon bundt ring, from mix	1/16 cake	290	270
lemon chiffon, from mix	1/12 cake	190	190
lemon pudding, from mix	1/6 cake	270	230
lemon, from mix	1/12 cake	260	220
marble streusel, w/icing, from mix	2.3 oz	278	224
marble, from mix	1/10 cake	280	270
w/white icing	1.8 oz	129	165
orange			
from mix	1/12 cake	280	260
homemade, w/icing	1.8 oz	141	183
pineapple upside-down			
from mix	1/9 cake	215	270
homemade	2.6 oz	179	236
plum pudding, canned	3.6 oz	150	270
pound			
commercial	1.1 lb loaf	1,857	1,935
	1 oz	108	110
from mix	1/12 cake	155	200
homemade	1.1 lb loaf	1,645	2,025
	1 oz	96	120
sheet, plain, homemade, w/ vegetable oil			
unfrosted	whole (9" square)	2,331	2,830
	1/9 cake	258	315
w/uncooked white icing	whole (9" square)	2,488	4,020
	1/9 cake	275	445
w/blackberries	5.2 oz	105	347
snack cake, small, commercial			
devil's food w/cream filling	1 oz	105	105
sponge w/cream filling	1½ oz	155	155
sour cream, from mix	1/8 cake	235	270
chocolate	1/12 cake	420	260
white	1/12 cake	260	180
spice, from mix	1.8 oz	175	175
w/vanilla icing	1.8 oz	193	176
sponge, homemade	2.3 oz	164	188
strawberry, from mix	1/12 cake	300	260
streusel swirl, from mix	1/16 cake	235	263

	Portion	Sodium (mg)	Calories
white			
from mix	2½ oz	293	219
homemade	2.7 oz	346	285
white, w/chocolate icing, homemade	2.7 oz	219	298
white, w/white icing, commercial	whole, 2-layer (8″ or 9″ diam)	2,827	4,170
	¹⁄₁₆ cake	176	260
yellow, homemade	2.6 oz	379	283
yellow, w/chocolate icing			
commercial	whole, 2-layer (8″ or 9″ diam)	3,080	3,895
	¹⁄₁₆ cake	192	245
from mix	whole, 2-layer (8″ or 9″ diam)	2,515	3,735
	¹⁄₁₆ cake	157	235
homemade	2.6 oz	208	292
yellow cupcake, w/vanilla icing	1.4 oz	184	160

Cake Icing

	Portion	Sodium (mg)	Calories
caramel	1.4 oz	35	140
chocolate	1.4 oz	23	148
chocolate fudge	1.4 oz	70	150
chocolate, double dark	1.3 oz	80	150
coconut	1.4 oz	47	140
coconut almond	1.2 oz	95	170
coconut pecan	1.2 oz	105	150
lemon	1.2 oz	15	140
milk chocolate	1.1 oz	55	150
strawberry	1.1 oz	55	140
vanilla	1.3 oz	30	150
white, fluffy	0.6 oz	85	70

Danish, Doughnuts, Sweet Rolls, & Toaster Pastries

	Portion	Sodium (mg)	Calories
danish pastry			
plain, w/out fruit or nuts	12 oz ring	1,302	1,305
	1 (4¼″ diam)	218	220
	1 oz	109	110
cinnamon raisin, from refrigerator dough	2.7 oz	450	270
fruit	1 round	233	235
doughnut			
cake type, plain	1.8 oz	192	210
yeast-leavened, glazed	2.1 oz	222	235

	Portion	Sodium (mg)	Calories
sweet roll	1	170	154
cinnamon w/icing, from refrigerator dough	2	517	230
toaster pastries	1	91	210

Fruit Bettys, Cobblers, Crisps, & Turnovers

	Portion	Sodium (mg)	Calories
apple brown Betty	½ c	214	211
apple crisp	½ c	228	302
apple dumpling	1	210	280
peach cobbler	⅓ c	158	160
peach crisp	½ c	235	249
turnover, from mix, apple, blueberry, or cherry	1	307	173

Pastry

	Portion	Sodium (mg)	Calories
éclair			
w/chocolate icing & custard filling	1	82	239
w/chocolate icing & whipped cream filling	3.7 oz	49	296
cream puff, w/custard filling	1 cream puff	108	303
pastry shells & pie crusts *See* BAKING INGREDIENTS			

Pie

	Portion	Sodium (mg)	Calories
apple, w/vegetable shortening crust	whole (9″ diam)	2,844	2,420
	⅙ pie	476	405
banana custard, homemade	⅛ pie	221	252
blackberry, homemade	⅛ pie	316	287
blueberry, w/vegetable shortening crust	whole (9″ diam)	2,533	2,285
	⅙ pie	423	380
butterscotch, homemade	⅛ pie	244	304
cherry, w/vegetable shortening crust	whole (9″ diam)	2,893	2,465
	⅙ pie	480	410
chocolate chiffon, homemade	⅛ pie	204	266
chocolate cream, homemade	4 oz	311	301
coconut custard, homemade	⅛ pie	282	268
cream, w/vegetable shortening crust	whole (9″ diam)	2,207	2,710
	⅙ pie	369	455
custard, w/vegetable shortening crust	whole (9″ diam)	2,612	1,985
	⅙ pie	436	330
fried			
apple	3 oz	326	255
cherry	3 oz	371	250

	Portion	Sodium (mg)	Calories
lemon chiffon, homemade	⅛ pie	211	254
lemon meringue, w/vegetable shortening crust	whole (9″ diam)	2,369	2,140
	⅙ pie	395	355
mincemeat, homemade	⅛ pie	529	320
peach, w/vegetable shortening crust	whole (9″ diam)	2,533	2,410
	⅙ pie	423	405
pecan, w/vegetable shortening crust	whole (9″ diam)	1,823	3,450
	⅙ pie	305	575
pumpkin, w/vegetable shortening crust	whole (9″ diam)	1,947	1,920
	⅙ pie	325	320
raisin, homemade	⅛ pie	336	319
rhubarb, homemade	⅛ pie	319	299
strawberry, homemade	⅛ pie	180	184
sweet potato, homemade	⅛ pie	249	243

Pie Fillings *See* DESSERTS: CUSTARDS, GELATINS, PUDDINGS, & PIE FILLINGS

▪ BRAND NAME

Dromedary

date nut roll	½″ slice	160	80

Kellogg's
POP-TARTS

blueberry	1	220	210
brown sugar cinnamon	1	210	210

FROSTED POP-TARTS

blueberry	1	220	200
brown sugar cinnamon	1	200	210
chocolate fudge	1	230	200
Dutch apple	1	210	210
peanut butter & jelly	1	220	220

Nabisco

Frosted Toastettes or Toastettes, all flavors	1	170–220	200

Pepperidge Farm Frozen Cakes & Pastries
FRUIT SQUARES

apple	1	170	220
blueberry	1	190	220
cherry	1	180	230

	Portion	Sodium (mg)	Calories
LAYER CAKES			
coconut	1⅝ oz	120	180
devil's food	1⅝ oz	140	170
German chocolate	1⅝ oz	170	180
golden	1⅝ oz	110	180
vanilla	1⅝ oz	120	190
OLD FASHIONED CAKES			
butter pound	1 oz	150	130
carrot w/cream cheese icing	1⅜ oz	150	140
PUFF PASTRY			
apple dumplings	3 oz	230	260
patty shells	1	180	210
puff pastry sheets	¼ sheet	290	260
turnovers			
apple	1	210	300
blueberry	1	240	320
cherry	1	290	310
peach	1	260	320
raspberry	1	270	320
SUPREME CAKES			
Boston cream	2⅞ oz	190	290
chocolate	2⅞ oz	140	310
lemon coconut	3 oz	220	280
raspberry mocha	3⅛ oz	170	310
strawberry cream	2 oz	120	190
Pillsbury			
SWEET ROLLS			
Best apple danish w/icing	1	260	240
Best quick cinnamon rolls w/ icing	1	260	210
cinnamon raisin danish w/icing	2	450	290
cinnamon rolls w/icing	2	520	230
TURNOVERS			
apple	1	320	170
blueberry or cherry	1	310	170
Rich's			
Bavarian cream puffs	1	66	150
chocolate éclairs	2 oz	113	210
Sara Lee			
ALL BUTTER COFFEE CAKES			
butter streusel	⅛ cake	160	160

	Portion	Sodium (mg)	Calories
cheese	⅛ cake	210	210
pecan	⅛ cake	180	160

ALL BUTTER POUND CAKES

Original	⅒ cake	85	130
Family Size	1/15 cake	85	130

INDIVIDUAL DANISH

apple	1	120	120
cheese	1	130	130
cinnamon raisin	1	140	150

LIGHT CLASSICS

chocolate mousse cake	⅒ pkg	80	200
French cheesecake			
plain	⅒ pkg	100	200
strawberry	⅒ pkg	100	200

SINGLE-LAYER ICED CAKES

banana	⅛ cake	160	170
carrot	⅛ cake	240	260

TWO-LAYER CAKES

Black Forest	⅛ cake	100	190
strawberry shortcake	⅛ cake	90	190

❑ DESSERTS: CUSTARDS, GELATINS, PUDDINGS, & PIE FILLINGS

Custard

plain			
baked, homemade	½ c	104	153
boiled, homemade	½ c	103	164
from mix	½ c	219	161
banana	½ c	125	143
chocolate	½ c	153	142
coconut	½ c	124	144
lemon	½ c	92	143
vanilla	½ c	128	143

Gelatin

Bavarian (w/whipped cream)			
chocolate	1 serving	103	347
strawberry	1 serving	79	277
made w/water, all flavors	½ c	54	81

	Portion	Sodium (mg)	Calories
Pie Filling			
pumpkin pie mix, canned	½ c	280	141
Pudding			
chocolate			
canned	5 oz	285	205
from mix, prepared w/whole milk			
regular	½ c	167	150
instant	½ c	440	155
rice w/raisins, homemade	½ c	94	194
rice, from mix, prepared w/ whole milk	½ c	140	155
tapioca			
canned	5 oz	252	160
from mix, prepared w/whole milk	½ c	152	145
homemade	½ c	257	111
vanilla			
canned	5 oz	305	220
from mix, prepared w/whole milk			
regular	½ c	178	145
instant	½ c	375	150
homemade	½ c	166	142
Rennin Dessert			
plain, homemade	½ c	104	113
chocolate, from mix			
prepared w/whole milk	½ c	59	127
prepared w/skim milk	½ c	63	95
fruit vanilla, from mix			
prepared w/whole milk	½ c	65	140
prepared w/skim milk	½ c	58	88
▪ BRAND NAME			
D-Zerta			
gelatin, low-cal	½ c	0	8
pudding, reduced-calorie, prepared w/skim milk			
chocolate	½ c	70	60
vanilla	½ c	65	70
Featherweight			
custard, lemon or vanilla	½ c	40	40
gelatin, low-sodium, low-cal			
cherry or lemon	½ c	4	10

	Portion	Sodium (mg)	Calories
gelatin, low sodium, low-cal *(cont.)*			
lime or orange	½ c	5	10
raspberry or strawberry	½ c	3	10
mousse, low-cal, chocolate	½ c	35	85
pudding			
butterscotch or vanilla	½ c	6	12
chocolate	½ c	15	12

Jell-O
AMERICANA DESSERTS, PREPARED W/WHOLE MILK

golden egg custard	½ c	200	160
rice pudding	½ c	160	170
tapioca pudding			
chocolate	½ c	170	170
vanilla	½ c	170	160

GELATIN

black raspberry or concord grape	½ c	35	80
cherry	½ c	70	80
lemon or wild strawberry	½ c	75	80
lime	½ c	55	80
orange-pineapple	½ c	65	80
all others	½ c	50	80

PUDDING & PIE FILLING
Regular, Prepared w/Whole Milk

butterscotch	½ c	190	170
chocolate	½ c	170	160
vanilla	½ c	200	160

Instant, Prepared w/Whole Milk

banana cream	½ c	440	160
butterscotch	½ c	480	160
chocolate	½ c	520	180
lemon	½ c	400	170
vanilla	½ c	440	170

Sugar-free Instant, Prepared w/2% Low-Fat Milk

banana	½ c	430	90
butterscotch	½ c	420	90
chocolate	½ c	410	100
vanilla	½ c	420	90

Sugar-free, Prepared w/2% Low-Fat Milk

chocolate	½ c	170	90
vanilla	½ c	200	80

	Portion	Sodium (mg)	Calories
RICH & DELICIOUS MOUSSE, PREPARED W/WHOLE MILK			
chocolate or chocolate fudge	½ c	85	150
Rich's Puddings			
butterscotch	3 oz	128	133
chocolate	3 oz	136	141
vanilla	3 oz	162	129
Royal			
GELATIN			
all flavors			
regular	½ c	90–100	80
sugar-free	½ c	70–75	6
PUDDING & PIE FILLING			
Cooked			
banana cream, prepared	½ c	210	160
butterscotch, prepared	½ c	210	160
chocolate			
dry	0.9 oz	90	120
prepared	½ c	150	180
custard, prepared	½ c	115	150
Dark 'n Sweet, prepared	½ c	150	180
flan w/caramel sauce, prepared	½ c	115	150
key lime, prepared	½ c	120	160
lemon			
dry	½ oz	100	50
prepared	½ c	120	160
vanilla			
dry	0.7 oz	150	80
prepared	½ c	210	160
Instant			
banana cream or butterscotch, prepared	½ c	390	180
chocolate			
dry	1 oz	330	120
prepared	½ c	390	190
Dark 'n Sweet, prepared	½ c	390	190
lemon			
dry	0.8 oz	290	110
prepared	½ c	350	180
pistachio nut, prepared	½ c	350	170
vanilla			
dry	0.8 oz	330	100
prepared	½ c	390	180
Instant Sugar-free			
butterscotch, prepared	½ c	470	100

	Portion	Sodium (mg)	Calories
chocolate			
dry	½ oz	420	50
prepared	½ c	480	110
vanilla			
dry	0.4 oz	410	40
prepared	½ c	470	100

❑ DESSERTS, FROZEN: ICE CREAM, ICE MILK, ICES & SHERBETS, & FROZEN JUICE, PUDDING, TOFU, & YOGURT

Frozen Pudding on a Stick

banana	1	63	94
butterscotch	1	63	94
chocolate	1	103	99
chocolate fudge	1	105	99
vanilla	1	63	93

Frozen Yogurt on a Stick

plain	1	15	65
carob/chocolate-coated	1	15	135

Ice Cream

chocolate	1 c	75	295
French custard	1 c	84	257
French vanilla, soft serve	1 c	153	377
strawberry	1 c	59	250
vanilla			
16% fat	1 c	108	349
10% fat	1 c	116	269

Ice Cream Novelties & Cones

ice cream cone (cone only)	1	28	45
ice cream sandwich	1	92	167
vanilla ice cream bar w/chocolate coating	1	28	162
vanilla ice milk bar w/chocolate coating	1	38	144

Ice Milk

chocolate	⅔ c	61	137
strawberry	⅔ c	64	133

	Portion	Sodium (mg)	Calories
vanilla			
regular	1 c	105	184
soft serve	1 c	162	223

Ices & Sherbets

	Portion	Sodium (mg)	Calories
lime/orange ice	1 c	tr	247
	⅔ c	tr	165
orange sherbet	1 c	88	270

▪ BRAND NAME

Baskin-Robbins
CONES

sugar	1	45	57
waffle	1	5	140

ICE CREAM & SHERBET

chocolate	1 regular scoop	160	270
chocolate chip	1 regular scoop	110	260
French vanilla	1 regular scoop	90	280
Jamoca Almond Fudge	1 regular scoop	115	270
Pralines 'n Cream	1 regular scoop	180	280
rainbow sherbet	1 regular scoop	85	160
red raspberry sorbet	1 regular scoop	25	140
Rocky Road	1 regular scoop	135	300
vanilla	1 regular scoop	115	240
Very Berry Strawberry	1 regular scoop	95	220

Ben & Jerry's Ice Cream

Cherry Garcia	4 fl oz	75	280
chocolate	4 fl oz	47	290
Chunky Monkey	4 fl oz	81	319
Heath Bar Crunch	4 fl oz	114	310
mint w/Oreo cookies	4 fl oz	131	296
vanilla	4 fl oz	71	267
Vanilla Chocolate Chunk	4 fl oz	79	304
White Russian	4 fl oz	67	271

	Portion	Sodium (mg)	Calories
Comet			
cups	1	5	20
sugar cones	1	35	40
Dole			
FRESH LITE BARS			
cherry or raspberry	1	6	25
lemon	1	16	25
pineapple-orange	1	7	25
FRUIT & CREAM BARS			
blueberry	1	20	90
FRUIT & CREAM BARS			
blueberry	1	20	90
chocolate-banana	1	20	175
chocolate-strawberry	1	20	140
peach	1	19	90
raspberry	1	23	90
strawberry	1	22	90
FRUIT & YOGURT BARS			
cherry	1	22	80
raspberry	1	18	70
strawberry	1	16	70
FRUIT 'N JUICE BARS			
piña colada	1	2	90
FRUIT 'N JUICE BARS			
piña colada	1	2	90
pineapple	1	4	70
raspberry	1	14	70
strawberry	1	6	70
SORBETS			
mandarin orange	4 oz	9	110
peach	4 oz	11	120
pineapple	4 oz	11	120
raspberry	4 oz	12	110
strawberry	4 oz	11	110

	Portion	Sodium (mg)	Calories
SUN TOP BARS			
fruit punch, grape, lemonade, or tropical orange	1	5	40
Drumstick			
Drumstick sundae cone	1	57	186
Häagen-Dazs			
ICE CREAM			
butter pecan	4 fl oz	95	290
chocolate	4 fl oz	50	270
chocolate chocolate chip	4 fl oz	40	290
coffee or vanilla	4 fl oz	55	260
honey vanilla	4 fl oz	55	250
key lime sorbet & vanilla	4 fl oz	35	200
macadamia nut	4 fl oz	80	330
orange sorbet & vanilla	4 fl oz	30	200
raspberry sorbet & vanilla	4 fl oz	30	180
rum raisin	4 fl oz	45	250
strawberry	4 fl oz	40	250
vanilla Swiss almond	4 fl oz	55	290
ICE CREAM BARS			
chocolate w/dark chocolate coating	1	60	390
vanilla w/dark chocolate coating	1	65	390
vanilla w/milk chocolate coating	1	55	360
vanilla w/milk chocolate coating & almonds	1	55	370
Jell-O			
FRUIT BARS			
all flavors	1	10	45
GELATIN POPS			
all flavors	1	5	35
PUDDING POPS			
chocolate	1	80	80
chocolate-covered vanilla	1	50	130
vanilla w/chocolate chips	1	50	80

	Portion	Sodium (mg)	Calories
Life Savers			
Flavor Pops, all flavors	1	0	40
Minute Maid Frozen Fruit Juice Bars			
Snack Pack	1 oz	5	25
Oreo Cookies 'n Cream			
ICE CREAM			
chocolate	3 fl oz	100	140
vanilla	3 fl oz	100	140
NOVELTIES			
on a stick	1	100	220
sandwich	1	300	240
Snackwich	1	80	60
Popsicle			
Creamsicle	1	27	103
Fudgsicle	1	55	91
Tofutti			
all flavors	4 oz	65–130	90–230
PINTS			
Cappuccino Love Drops	4 fl oz	120	230
Chocolate Love Drops	4 fl oz	100	230
Chocolate Supreme	4 fl oz	130	210
vanilla	4 fl oz	90	200
vanilla almond bark	4 fl oz	95	230
Vanilla Love Drops	4 fl oz	100	220
wildberry	4 fl oz	100	210
SINGLE SERVINGS			
Chocolate Cuties	1	130	140
Vanilla Cuties	1	110	130
SOFT SERVE			
Lite-Lite			
chocolate	4 fl oz	80	100
vanilla	4 fl oz	80	90
regular	4 fl oz	65	158

❑ DESSERT SAUCES, SYRUPS, & TOPPINGS

See also NUTS & NUT-BASED BUTTERS, FLOURS,
MEALS, MILKS, PASTES, & POWDERS

	Portion	Sodium (mg)	Calories
Sauces, Syrups, & Flavored Toppings			
butterscotch topping	3 T	111	156
caramel topping	3 T	152	155
cherry topping	3 T	17	147
chocolate-flavored syrup or topping			
fudge type	2 T	42	125
thin type	2 T	36	85
honey *See* SUGARS & SWEETENERS			
pineapple topping	3 T	17	146
walnuts in syrup topping	3 T	tr	169
Whipped Cream & Whipped Cream–Type Toppings			
nondairy			
powdered, prepared w/whole	1 T	3	8
milk	1 c	53	151
pressurized, containing lauric	1 T	2	11
acid oil & sodium caseinate	1 c	43	184
semisolid, frozen, containing	1 T	1	13
lauric acid oil & sodium caseinate	1 c	19	239
whipped cream topping, pres-	1 T	4	8
surized	1 c	78	154

- **BRAND NAME**

	Portion	Sodium (mg)	Calories
Cool Whip			
Extra Creamy Dairy Recipe whipped topping	1 T	0	16
nondairy whipped topping	1 T	0	12
D-Zerta			
reduced-calorie whipped top- ping	1 T	5	8
Dream Whip			
whipped topping mix, prepared w/whole milk	1 T	0	10
Featherweight			
whipped topping	1 T	5	4
Hershey			
chocolate fudge topping	2 T	30	100

	Portion	Sodium (mg)	Calories
Smucker's			
butterscotch	2 T	75	140
caramel	2 T	110	140
chocolate fudge	2 T	45	130
fruit syrups	2 T	0	100
hot caramel	2 T	75	150
hot fudge	2 T	55	110
peanut butter caramel	2 T	105	150
pineapple	2 T	0	130
strawberry	2 T	0	120
walnuts in syrup	2 T	0	130

❑ DINNERS, FROZEN

▪ BRAND NAME

	Portion	Sodium (mg)	Calories
Hungry-Man Dinners *See* Swanson, *below*			
Le Menu			
beef sirloin tips	11½ oz	780	400
beef Stroganoff	10 oz	1,100	450
chicken à la king	10¼ oz	810	330
chicken cordon bleu	11 oz	870	470
chicken Florentine	12½ oz	990	340
chicken parmigiana	11½ oz	900	400
chopped sirloin beef	12¼ oz	1,030	440
ham steak	10 oz	1,490	300
pepper steak	11½ oz	1,030	370
sliced breast of turkey w/mushroom gravy	10½ oz	1,020	270
sweet & sour chicken	11¼ oz	1,170	450
Yankee pot roast	11 oz	780	370
Le Menu Light Style			
chicken cacciatore	10 oz	640	270
glazed chicken breast	10 oz	770	270
Salisbury steak	10½ oz	830	220
3-cheese stuffed shells	10 oz	720	280
turkey divan	10 oz	840	280
veal Marsala	10 oz	800	260
Swanson			
3-COMPARTMENT DINNERS			
beans & franks	10½ oz	900	440

	Portion	Sodium (mg)	Calories
macaroni & beef	12 oz	870	370
macaroni & cheese	12¼ oz	990	260
noodles & chicken	10½ oz	860	270
spaghetti & meatballs	12½ oz	1,010	370

4-COMPARTMENT DINNERS

beef	11¼ oz	800	340
beef enchiladas	13¾ oz	1,300	480
beef in barbecue sauce	11 oz	850	460
chicken in barbecue sauce	11¾ oz	940	460
chicken nugget platter	8¾ oz	710	460
chopped sirloin beef	11 oz	850	370
fish & chips	10 oz	930	500
fish nugget	9½ oz	930	410
fried chicken			
barbecue-flavored	edible portion = 10 oz	1,000	520
dark meat	edible portion = 10 oz	1,100	560
white meat	edible portion = 10½ oz	1,380	560
loin of pork	10¾ oz	770	310
meat loaf	10¾ oz	1,030	430
Mexican-style combination	14¼ oz	1,580	520
Salisbury steak	10¾ oz	880	410
sweet & sour chicken	12 oz	520	380
Swiss steak	10 oz	740	340
turkey	11½ oz	1,110	350
veal parmigiana	12¼ oz	1,100	450
Western style	11½ oz	1,010	450

HUNGRY-MAN DINNERS

boneless chicken	17¾ oz	1,530	700
chopped beef steak	16¾ oz	1,600	640
fried chicken			
dark meat	14¼ oz	1,660	860
white meat	14¼ oz	2,150	870
Mexican style	20¼ oz	2,080	820
Salisbury steak	18¼ oz	1,730	680
sliced beef	15¼ oz	1,060	450
turkey	17 oz	1,810	550
veal parmigiana	18¼ oz	2,080	560

	Portion	Sodium (mg)	Calories

❏ EGGS & EGG SUBSTITUTES

Chicken Eggs

COOKED

egg dishes, prepared *See* BREAKFAST FOODS, PREPARED; FAST FOODS

	Portion	Sodium (mg)	Calories
fried in butter	1 large	144	83
hard boiled	1 large	69	79
omelet, cooked w/butter & MILK	1 egg (large)	155	95
poached	1 large	146	79
scrambled, w/butter & milk	1 large	155	95

DRIED

whole	1 c sifted	443	505
whole, stabilized (glucose-reduced)	1 c sifted	466	523
white only			
flakes, stabilized (glucose-reduced)	½ lb	2,622	796
powder, stabilized (glucose-reduced)	1 c sifted	1,325	402
yolk only	1 c sifted	61	460

UNCOOKED

whole, fresh or frozen	1	69	79
white only, fresh or frozen	1	50	16
yolk only, fresh	1	8	63

Eggs, Other

duck	1	102	130

Egg Substitute

frozen, containing egg white, corn oil, & nonfat dry milk	¼ c	120	96
liquid, containing egg white, soybean oil, & soy protein	1 c	444	211
powder, containing egg white solids, whole egg solids, sweet whey solids, nonfat dry milk, & soy protein	0.7 oz	158	88

	Portion	Sodium (mg)	Calories
■ BRAND NAME			
Featherweight			
egg substitute	2 eggs	247	120
Fleischmann's			
Egg Beaters	¼ c	80	25
Egg Beaters w/Cheez	½ c	440	130

❑ ENTREES & MAIN COURSES, CANNED & BOXED

chili & bean products, canned & boxed *See* LEGUMES & LEGUME PRODUCTS; SOYBEANS & SOYBEAN PRODUCTS

	Portion	Sodium (mg)	Calories
■ BRAND NAME			
Armour Star			
beef stew	8 oz	1,320	220
corned & roast beef hash & sloppy joes *See* PROCESSED MEAT & POULTRY PRODUCTS			
Chun King			
DIVIDER PAK ENTREES, CANNED			
2 Servings/24 Oz Pkg			
beef chow mein	8 oz	640	110
chicken chow mein	8 oz	940	120
4 Servings/42 Oz Pkg			
beef chow mein	7 oz	560	100
beef pepper Oriental	7 oz	880	110
chicken chow mein	7 oz	820	110
pork chow mein	7 oz	500	120
shrimp chow mein	7 oz	260	100
STIR-FRY ENTREES, CANNED			
chow mein w/beef	6 oz	540	290
chow mein w/chicken	6 oz	540	220
egg foo young	5 oz	520	140
pepper steak	6 oz	1,000	250
sukiyaki	6 oz	400	260
Featherweight			
beef ravioli	8 oz	75	220
beef stew	7½ oz	390	160
boned chicken	3 oz	38	186
chicken stew	7½ oz	55	170
chicken w/dumplings	7½ oz	115	160
spaghetti w/meatballs	7½ oz	95	200

	Portion	Sodium (mg)	Calories
Franco-American			
beef ravioli in meat sauce	7½ oz	920	250
macaroni & cheese	7⅜ oz	960	170
spaghetti in tomato sauce w/cheese	7⅜ oz	810	190
spaghetti w/meatballs in tomato sauce	7⅜ oz	850	220
SpaghettiO's in tomato & cheese sauce	7⅜ oz	920	170
Noodle-Roni Pasta			
chicken & mushroom flavor, prepared	1.2 oz	550	160
creamy garlic, prepared	1½ oz	630	300
fettucini, prepared	1½ oz	560	300
herbs & butter, prepared	1 oz	290	160
parmesano, prepared	1.2 oz	470	240
pesto Italiano, prepared	1.2 oz	340	220
Rominoff, prepared	1½ oz	730	240
Stroganoff, prepared	2 oz	1,190	350
Swanson			
chicken & dumplings	7½ oz	960	220
chicken à la king	5¼ oz	690	180
chicken stew	7⅝ oz	960	170
Van Camp's			
Noodle Weenee	1 c	12	245
tamales w/sauce	1 c	1,132	293

❑ ENTREES & MAIN COURSES, FROZEN

	Portion	Sodium (mg)	Calories
Celentano			
baked pasta & cheese	6 oz	350	290
broccoli stuffed shells	6¾ oz	360	231
cannelloni Florentine	12 oz	540	380
cavatelli	3.2 oz	100	270
chicken cutlets parmigiana	9 oz	750	310
chicken primavera	11½ oz	650	270
eggplant parmigiana	7 oz	330	270
	8 oz	405	330
	10 oz	500	350
Eggplant Rollettes	11 oz	510	420
lasagne	8 oz	410	320
	10 oz	870	460
lasagne primavera	11 oz	500	300
manicotti			
w/sauce	8 oz	435	300
	10 oz	860	380
w/out sauce	7 oz	420	380

	Portion	Sodium (mg)	Calories
ravioli			
miniround cheese, w/out sauce	4 oz	180	250
round cheese, w/out sauce	6½ oz	360	410
stuffed shells			
w/sauce	8 oz	425	320
	10 oz	850	410
w/out sauce	6¼ oz	265	350
stuffed sweet red peppers	12½ oz	530	290
Contadina Fresh Refrigerated Filled Pasta			
agnolotti	4.5 oz	340	380
EGG			
ravioli w/cheese	4.5 oz	640	410
ravioli w/meat	4.5 oz	540	380
tortellini w/cheese	4.5 oz	570	380
tortellini w/chicken & prosciutto	4.5 oz	560	370
tortellini w/meat	4.5 oz	580	380
SPINACH			
ravioli w/cheese	4.5 oz	660	400
tortellini w/cheese	4.5 oz	590	380
tortellini w/meat	4.5 oz	610	380
Le Menu Entrees			
beef burgundy	7½ oz	660	330
chicken Kiev	8 oz	780	530
manicotti	8½ oz	1,030	410
Oriental chicken	10½ oz	820	330
Mrs. Paul's			
eggplant parmigiana *See* VEGETABLES, PLAIN & PREPARED			
AU NATUREL SEAFOOD			
cod fillets	5 oz	200	110
flounder fillets	5 oz	210	110
haddock fillets	5 oz	230	100
perch fillets	5 oz	200	110
sole fillets	5 oz	170	110
BUTTERED SEAFOOD			
fish fillets	2	390	170
LIGHT SEAFOOD ENTREES			
fish & pasta Florentine	9 oz	870	230
fish au gratin	9 oz	1,100	270
fish Dijon	8¾ oz	430	210
fish Florentine	8 oz	580	200
fish Mornay	9 oz	660	250

	Portion	Sodium (mg)	Calories
shrimp & clams w/linguini	10 oz	790	280
shrimp Cajun style	9 oz	860	200
shrimp primavera	9½ oz	980	190
tuna pasta casserole	10 oz	960	270

PREPARED BATTERED SEAFOOD

batter-dipped fish fillets	2	580	320
Crunchy Light Batter			
fish fillets	2	810	310
fish sticks	4	590	240
flounder fillets	2	810	310
haddock fillets	2	670	330
fried clams in a light batter	2½ oz	380	240

PREPARED BREADED SEAFOOD

catfish fillet strips	4 oz	290	240
combination seafood platter	9 oz	1,220	590
Crispy Crunchy			
fish fillets	2	550	280
fish sticks	4	350	200
flounder fillets	2	500	270
haddock fillets	2	410	280
ocean perch fillets	2	460	320
deviled crabs	1 piece	390	170
fish cakes	2	840	250
french-fried scallops	3½ oz	480	230
fried shrimp	3 oz	430	200
Supreme Light Breaded			
fish fillets	1	540	210

Sara Lee Le Sandwich Croissants

cheddar cheese	1	910	380
chicken & broccoli	1	600	340
ham & Swiss cheese	1	860	340
turkey, bacon, & cheese	1	895	370

Swanson
CHICKEN DUET ENTREES

creamy broccoli	6 oz	590	320
creamy green bean	6 oz	570	330
saucy tomato	6 oz	600	340
savory wild rice	6 oz	580	330

CHICKEN DUET GOURMET NUGGETS

ham & cheese	2.7 oz	370	190
Mexican style	2.7 oz	370	200
pizza style	2.7 oz	400	190
spinach & herb	2.7 oz	380	230

	Portion	Sodium (mg)	Calories
ENTREES			
Chicken Nibbles	edible portion = 4¼ oz	480	340
Fish 'n' Fries	6½ oz	690	350
fried chicken	edible portion = 7 oz	1,030	380
Salisbury steak	10 oz	1,170	480
Swedish meatballs	8½ oz	780	350
turkey w/dressing & potatoes	9 oz	1,020	290
veal parmigiana	10 oz	960	330
HUNGRY-MAN POT PIES			
beef	16 oz	1,530	700
chicken	16 oz	1,630	740
turkey	16 oz	1,670	750
MAIN COURSE ENTREES			
lasagna w/meat	10½ oz	870	400
macaroni & cheese	10 oz	980	400
PLUMP & JUICY			
Chicken Dipsters	3 oz	390	220
Chicken Drumlets	3 oz	370	220
Chicken Nibbles	3¼ oz	660	300
fried chicken, breast portions	4½ oz	770	360
Take-Out fried chicken, assorted pieces	3¼ oz	630	270
thighs & drumsticks	3¼ oz	550	280
POT PIES			
beef	7 oz	700	380
chicken	7 oz	810	370
macaroni & cheese	7 oz	880	220
turkey	7 oz	720	390

❑ FAST FOODS

	Portion	Sodium (mg)	Calories
shakes			
chocolate	10 fl oz	273	360
strawberry	10 fl oz	234	319
vanilla	10 fl oz	232	314
tacos	1	456	195

	Portion	Sodium (mg)	Calories
■ BRAND NAME			

Arby's
BEVERAGES

coffee	6 oz	2	2
milk, whole	8 oz	119	227
milk, 2% fat	8 oz	122	121
orange juice	6 oz	2	82

BREAKFAST ITEMS

biscuit			
bacon	1	960	330
ham	1	1,190	325
plain	1	730	280
sausage	1	1,000	460
cinnamon nut danish	1	230	340
croissant			
bacon/egg	1	580	469
ham & cheese	1	960	345
mushroom/cheese	1	625	337
plain	1	300	260
sausage/egg	1	619	600
French toast syrup	1½ oz	48	219
ham platter	1	1,192	719
sausage platter	1	841	816
Toastix	1	440	420

DESSERTS

apple turnover	1	178	303
cherry turnover	1	200	280

DRESSINGS & SAUCES

Arby's sauce	1 oz	227	30
blue cheese dressing	2½ oz	766	390
Buttermilk Ranch dressing	2½ oz	598	210
honey French dressing	2½ oz	532	350
Horsey sauce	1 oz	210	110
light Italian dressing	2 oz	255	25
Thousand Island dressing	2½ oz	576	345

MISCELLANEOUS

chocolate chip cookie	1	95	130
croutons	½ oz	155	59

SALADS

chef salad	1	720	210
garden salad	1	99	149
side salad	1	30	25

	Portion	Sodium (mg)	Calories
SANDWICHES			
Bac'n Cheddar Deluxe	1	1,672	526
Beef'n Cheddar	1	955	455
chicken breast	1	1,019	493
chicken cashew salad	1	1,140	590
Chicken Cordon Bleu	1	1,824	630
corned beef	1	1,440	400
fish fillet	1	994	537
ham & cheese	1	1,350	292
Philly Beef 'n Swiss	1	1,300	460
reuben	1	1,900	450
roast beef			
regular	1	588	353
junior	1	345	218
king	1	766	467
super	1	798	501
giant	1	908	531
roast chicken club	1	1,500	610
Steak Deluxe	1	460	800
Steak 'n Cheddar	1	960	640
Sub Deluxe	1	1,600	540
Turkey Deluxe	1	1,047	375
SHAKES			
chocolate	1	341	451
Jamocha	1	262	368
vanilla	1	281	330
SIDE DISHES			
Cheddar Fries	1 serving	454	399
Curly Fries	1 serving	167	337
french fries	1 serving	114	246
potato cakes	1 serving	397	204
Burger King			
BREAKFAST ITEMS			
Breakfast Croissan'wich	1	637	304
w/bacon	1	762	355
w/ham	1	987	335
w/sausage	1	1,042	538
French toast sticks	1 serving	498	499
Great Danish	1	288	500
scrambled egg platter	1	808	468
w/bacon	1	975	536
w/sausage	1	1,213	702
BURGERS & SANDWICHES			
bacon double cheeseburger	1	728	510
cheeseburger	1	651	317

	Portion	Sodium (mg)	Calories
Chicken Specialty	1	1,423	688
Ham & Cheese Specialty	1	1,534	471
hamburger	1	509	275
Whaler fish	1	592	488
Whopper	1	880	628
w/cheese	1	1,164	711
Whopper Jr.	1	486	322
w/cheese	1	628	364

CHICKEN

Chicken Tenders	6 pieces	636	204

DESSERTS

apple pie	1 slice	412	305

SALAD DRESSINGS

bacon bits	1 packet	1	16
bleu cheese	1 packet	600	300
croutons	1 packet	88	29
French	1 packet	690	280
house	1 packet	530	260
reduced-calorie Italian	1 packet	870	30
Thousand Island	1 packet	470	240

SALADS

chef salad	1	570	180
chicken salad	1	440	140
garden salad	1	125	92
side salad	1	20	20

SHAKES

chocolate	1 regular	202	320
syrup added	1 regular	225	374
vanilla	1 regular	205	321
syrup added	1 regular	213	334

SIDE DISHES

french fries	1 regular serving	160	227
onion rings	1 regular serving	665	274

Church's Fried Chicken
CHICKEN

breast	1	560	278
leg	1	286	147
thigh	1	448	306
wing-breast	1	583	303

	Portion	Sodium (mg)	Calories
SIDE DISHES			
corn, w/butter oil	1 ear	20	237
french fries, w/salt	1 regular serving	126	138
Hardee's			
BREAKFAST ITEMS			
bacon & egg biscuit	1	1,175	410
Big Country Breakfast bacon	1 serving	1,238	761
Big Country Breakfast ham	1 serving	2,263	665
Big Country Breakfast sausage	1 serving	1,820	849
Canadian Sunrise biscuit	1	1,121	482
cinnamon & raisin biscuit	1	346	276
country ham biscuit	1	1,038	323
egg	1	54	79
ham biscuit	1	1,112	300
Hash Rounds potatoes	1 serving	558	232
Rise 'n' Shine biscuit	1	521	257
sausage & egg biscuit	1	885	503
sausage biscuit	1	831	426
steak biscuit	1	1,096	508
BURGERS & SANDWICHES			
bacon cheeseburger	1	2,042	556
big deluxe burger	1	868	503
cheeseburger			
regular	1	745	327
¼ lb	1	1,095	511
chicken fillet	1	1,258	413
Fisherman's Fillet	1	861	510
hamburger	1	548	244
hot dog	1	796	285
hot ham & cheese	1	1,833	316
mushroom & Swiss burger	1	1,051	509
roast beef			
regular	1	966	312
big	1	1,434	440
turkey club	1	1,185	426
DESSERTS			
apple turnover	1	204	87
Big Cookie Treat	1	258	54
Cool Twist cone			
chocolate	1	108	162
vanilla	1	89	164

	Portion	Sodium (mg)	Calories
SALADS			
chef salad	1	788	309
garden salad, w/Thousand Island dressing	1	207	246
side salad	1	43	90
SHAKES			
chocolate	1	241	390
SIDE DISHES			
Chicken Stix	6 pieces	887	234
french fries	1 regular serving	78	197
	1 large serving	153	371
Jack-in-the-Box			
BREAKFAST ITEMS			
Breakfast Jack	1	871	307
grape jelly	1 serving	3	38
pancake platter	1	888	612
pancake syrup	1 serving	6	121
scrambled egg platter	1	1,188	662
BURGERS & SANDWICHES			
bacon cheeseburger	1	1,127	705
cheeseburger	1	746	325
Chicken Supreme	1	1,525	575
club pita, w/out sauce	1	931	277
hamburger	1	556	288
Hot Club Supreme	1	1,467	524
Jumbo Jack	1	733	584
w/cheese	1	1,090	677
Swiss & bacon burger	1	1,458	678
Ultimate Cheeseburger	1	1,176	942
CRESCENT ROLLS			
Canadian crescent	1	851	452
sausage crescent	1	1,012	584
Supreme crescent	1	1,053	547
DESSERTS			
cheesecake	1 piece	208	309
hot apple turnover	1	350	410
MEXICAN DISHES			
Beef Fajita Pita	1	384	278
guacamole	1 serving	130	55
salsa	1 serving	129	8
Super taco	1	765	288
taco	1	406	191

	Portion	Sodium (mg)	Calories
SALAD DRESSINGS			
bleu cheese	1 serving	459	131
buttermilk house	1 serving	347	181
reduced-calorie French	1 serving	300	80
Thousand Island	1 serving	350	156
SALADS			
chef salad	1	900	325
side salad	1	84	51
taco salad	1	1,670	641
SAUCES			
BBQ	1 serving	300	44
Mayo-Mustard	1 serving	247	124
Mayo-Onion	1 serving	140	143
Seafood Cocktail	1 serving	206	33
SHAKES			
chocolate	1	270	330
strawberry	1	240	320
vanilla	1	230	320
SIDE DISHES			
french fries	1 regular serving	164	221
	1 large serving	262	353
onion rings	1 serving	407	382
Kentucky Fried Chicken			
FRIED CHICKEN			
Extra Crispy			
breast			
center	1	842	353
side	1	797	354
drumstick	1	346	173
thigh	1	766	371
wing	1	437	218
Original Recipe			
breast			
center	1	532	257
side	1	654	276
drumstick	1	269	147
thigh	1	517	278
wing	1	387	181
NUGGETS & SAUCES			
barbecue sauce	1 oz	450	35
honey sauce	½ oz	<15	49

	Portion	Sodium (mg)	Calories
mustard sauce	1 oz	346	36
nuggets	1	140	46
sweet & sour sauce	1 oz	148	58

SIDE DISHES

baked beans	1 serving	387	105
buttermilk biscuits	1	521	269
chicken gravy	1 serving	398	59
cole slaw	1 serving	171	103
corn on the cob	1 ear	<21	176
Kentucky fries	1 serving	81	268
mashed potatoes	1 serving	228	59
w/gravy	1 serving	297	62
potato salad	1 serving	396	141

McDonald's
BREAKFAST ITEMS

biscuit			
w/bacon, cheese, & egg	1	1,230	449
w/biscuit spread	1	730	260
w/sausage	1	1,080	440
w/sausage & egg	1	1,250	529
danish			
apple	1	370	389
cinnamon raisin	1	430	445
iced cheese	1	420	395
raspberry	1	310	414
Egg McMuffin	1	740	293
English muffin w/butter	1	270	169
hash brown potatoes	1 serving	330	131
hotcakes w/butter syrup	1 serving	640	413
pork sausage	1 serving	350	180
Sausage McMuffin	1	830	372
w/egg	1	980	451
scrambled eggs	1 serving	290	157

BURGERS & SANDWICHES

Big Mac	1	950	562
cheeseburger	1	750	308
Filet-o-Fish	1	1,030	442
hamburger	1	460	257
McD.L.T.	1	1,170	674
Quarter Pounder	1	660	414
w/cheese	1	1,150	517

CHICKEN NUGGETS & SAUCES

barbecue sauce	1 serving	340	53
Chicken McNuggets	2	520	288
honey	1 serving	0	46
hot mustard sauce	1 serving	250	66
sweet & sour sauce	1 serving	190	57

	Portion	Sodium (mg)	Calories
DESSERTS			
apple pie	1 piece	240	262
cookies			
Chocolaty Chip	1 serving	280	325
McDonaldland	1 serving	300	288
soft-serve ice cream & cone	1 serving	70	144
sundaes			
hot caramel	1	160	343
hot fudge	1	160	313
strawberry	1	85	283
SALAD BAR ITEMS			
bacon bits	1 serving	95	16
chef salad	1	490	231
chicken salad Oriental	1	230	141
chow mein noodles	1 serving	60	45
croutons	1 serving	140	52
garden salad	1	160	112
shrimp salad	1	480	104
side salad	1	85	57
SALAD DRESSINGS			
bleu cheese	½ oz	150	69
French	½ oz	180	58
lite vinaigrette	½ oz	60	15
Oriental	½ oz	180	24
Thousand Island	½ oz	100	78
SHAKES			
chocolate	1	240	388
strawberry	1	170	384
vanilla	1	170	354
SIDE DISHES			
french fries	1 regular serving	110	220
Pizza Hut			
HAND-TOSSED PIZZA			
cheese	2 slices	1,276	518
pepperoni	2 slices	1,267	500
Supreme	2 slices	1,490	540
Super Supreme	2 slices	1,648	556
PAN PIZZA			
cheese	2 slices	940	492
pepperoni	2 slices	1,127	540
Supreme	2 slices	1,363	589
Super Supreme	2 slices	1,447	563

	Portion	Sodium (mg)	Calories
PERSONAL PAN PIZZA			
pepperoni	2 slices	1,335	675
Supreme	2 slices	1,313	647
THIN 'N CRISPY PIZZA			
cheese	2 slices	867	398
pepperoni	2 slices	986	413
Supreme	2 slices	1,328	459
Super Supreme	2 slices	1,336	463
Roy Rogers			
BEVERAGES			
hot chocolate	1	125	123
BREAKFAST ITEMS			
crescent roll	1	547	287
crescent sandwich	1	867	401
w/bacon	1	1,035	431
w/ham	1	1,192	557
w/sausage	1	1,289	449
egg & biscuit platter	1	734	394
w/bacon	1	957	435
w/ham	1	1,156	442
w/sausage	1	1,059	550
pancake platter, w/syrup & butter	1	842	452
w/bacon	1	1,065	493
w/ham	1	1,264	506
w/sausage	1	1,167	608
BURGERS & SANDWICHES			
bacon cheeseburger	1	1,536	581
cheeseburger	1	1,404	563
hamburger	1	495	456
roast beef			
regular	1	785	317
w/cheese	1	1,694	424
large	1	1,044	360
w/cheese	1	1,953	467
RR Bar Burger	1	1,826	611
CHICKEN			
breast	1	509	412
breast & wing	1 each	894	604
drumstick/leg	1	190	140
nuggets	6	676	267
thigh	1	406	296
thigh & leg	1 each	596	436
wing	1	285	192

	Portion	Sodium (mg)	Calories
DESSERTS			
brownie	1	150	264
danish			
apple	1	255	249
cheese	1	260	254
cherry	1	242	271
strawberry shortcake	1 serving	674	447
sundaes			
caramel	1	193	293
hot fudge	1	186	337
strawberry	1	99	216
SALAD BAR ITEMS			
bacon bits	1 T	210	33
beets, sliced	¼ c	100	16
broccoli	½ c	7	20
carrots, shredded	¼ c	7	42
cheddar cheese	¼ c	195	112
Chinese noodles	¼ c	100	55
croutons	2 T	453	70
cucumbers	5–6 slices	2	4
eggs, chopped	2 T	41	55
green peas	¼ c	66	7
green peppers	¼ c	2	4
lettuce	1 c	7	10
macaroni salad	2 T	301	60
mushrooms	¼ c	3	5
potato salad	2 T	350	50
sunflower seeds	2 T	7	157
tomatoes	3 slices	3	20
SALAD DRESSINGS			
bacon & tomato	2 T	150	136
bleu cheese	2 T	153	150
low-cal Italian	2 T	100	70
Ranch	2 T	100	155
Thousand Island	2 T	150	160
SHAKES			
chocolate	1	290	358
strawberry	1	261	315
vanilla	1	282	306
SIDE DISHES			
biscuit	1	575	231
cole slaw	1 serving	261	110
french fries	1 regular serving	165	268
	1 large serving	221	357

	Portion	Sodium (mg)	Calories
hot topped potato			
plain	1	65	211
w/bacon & cheese	1	778	397
w/broccoli & cheese	1	523	376
w/oleo	1	161	274
w/sour cream & chives	1	138	408
w/taco beef & cheese	1	726	463
macaroni	1 serving	603	186
potato salad	1 serving	696	107
Wendy's			
BEVERAGES			
hot chocolate	1	120	110
lemonade	1	tr	160
BREAKFAST ITEMS			
bacon	1 strip	125	30
breakfast sandwich	1	770	370
buttermilk biscuit	1	860	320
danish			
apple	1	380	360
cheese	1	500	430
cinnamon raisin	1	430	410
French toast	2 slices	850	400
French toast toppings			
apple	1 pkt	120	130
blueberry	1 pkt	65	60
fried egg	1	95	90
grape jelly	1 pkt	tr	40
omelet #1: ham & cheese	1	570	290
omelet #2: ham, cheese, & mushroom	1	405	250
omelet #3: ham, cheese, onion, & green pepper	1	485	280
omelet #4: mushroom, green pepper, & onion	1	200	210
potatoes	1 serving	745	360
sausage gravy	6 oz	1,300	440
sausage patty	1	405	200
scrambled eggs	2 eggs	160	190
strawberry jam	1 pkt	tr	40
syrup	1 pkt	5	140
toast, w/margarine			
wheat	2 slices	315	190
white	2 slices	410	250
BURGER & SANDWICH COMPONENTS			
American cheese slice	1	295	60
bacon	1 strip	125	30

	Portion	Sodium (mg)	Calories
buns			
kaiser	1	390	180
multigrain	1	215	140
white	1	255	140
catsup	1 t	50	6
hamburger patty, ¼ lb	1	105	210
lettuce	1 leaf	tr	2
mayonnaise	1 T	60	90
mustard	1 t	45	4
onion	3 rings	tr	2
pickles, dill	4 slices	200	2
taco sauce	1 pkt	1,260	10
tartar sauce	1 T	75	80
tomatoes	1 slice	tr	2

BURGERS & SANDWICHES

	Portion	Sodium (mg)	Calories
Big Classic	1	900	470
chicken breast fillet	1	310	200
chicken fried steak	1	1,040	580
fish fillet	1	475	210
Kids' Meal hamburger	1	225	200

CHICKEN NUGGETS & SAUCES

	Portion	Sodium (mg)	Calories
barbecue sauce	1 pkt	100	50
Crispy Nuggets			
cooked in animal/vegetable oil	6	615	290
cooked in vegetable oil	6	660	310
honey	1 pkt	tr	45
sweet & sour sauce	1 pkt	55	45
sweet mustard sauce	1 pkt	140	50

CHILI

	Portion	Sodium (mg)	Calories
chili	1 regular serving	990	240

CONDIMENTS, SAUCES, & MISCELLANEOUS ITEMS

	Portion	Sodium (mg)	Calories
catsup	1 pkt	115	12
cheese sauce	2 oz	415	140
half & half	⅜ oz	5	14
hot chili seasoning	1 pkt	270	6
margarine			
liquid	½ oz	100	100
whipped	1 T	60	70
nondairy creamer	⅜ oz	10	14
saltines	2	70	25
sour cream	2 t	5	20
sugar	1 pkt	tr	14

	Portion	Sodium (mg)	Calories
DESSERTS			
chocolate chip cookie	1	235	320
Frosty dairy dessert	1 regular serving	220	400
SALAD BAR ITEMS			
alfalfa sprouts	1 oz	tr	8
American cheese	1 oz	365	90
bacon bits	⅛ oz	100	10
blueberries	1 T	tr	6
bread sticks	2	60	35
broccoli	½ c	5	12
cabbage, red	¼ c	5	4
cantaloupe	2 pieces	5	18
carrots	¼ c	15	10
cauliflower	½ c	5	12
celery	1 T	10	0
cheddar cheese	1 oz	310	80
cherry peppers	1 T	180	6
chow mein noodles	½ oz	105	70
cole slaw	¼ c	165	80
cottage cheese	½ c	425	110
croutons	½ oz	155	60
cucumbers	4 slices	tr	2
eggs	1 T	25	30
grapes	¼ c	tr	30
green peas	1 oz	35	25
green peppers	¼ c	5	8
honeydew melon	2 pieces	5	20
jalapeño peppers	1 T	4	9
lettuce			
iceberg	1 c	5	8
romaine	1 c	5	10
mozzarella cheese	1 oz	335	90
mushrooms	¼ c	tr	4
oranges	2 oz	0	25
Parmesan cheese, grated	1 oz	510	130
pasta salad	¼ c	190	130
peaches	2 slices	0	17
pepper rings	1 T	200	2
pineapple chunks	½ c	0	70
provolone cheese	1 oz	335	90
radishes	½ oz	tr	2
red onions	3 rings	tr	2
strawberries	2 oz	tr	18
sunflower seeds & raisins	1 oz	5	140
Swiss cheese	1 oz	365	90
tomatoes	1 oz	5	6
watermelon	2 pieces	tr	18

	Portion	Sodium (mg)	Calories
SALAD DRESSINGS			
Reduced-Calorie			
bacon/tomato	1 T	180	45
creamy cucumber	1 T	140	50
Italian	1 T	180	25
Thousand Island	1 T	125	45
Regular			
bleu cheese	1 T	85	60
celery seed	1 T	65	70
French style	1 T	130	70
Golden Italian	1 T	260	50
oil	1 T	0	120
Ranch	1 T	95	50
Thousand Island	1 T	115	70
wine vinegar	1 T	5	2
SIDE DISHES			
french fries			
cooked in animal/vegetable oil	1 regular serving	105	310
cooked in vegetable oil	1 regular serving	135	300
hot stuffed baked potatoes			
plain	1	60	250
bacon & cheese	1	1,180	570
broccoli & cheese	1	430	500
cheese	1	450	590
chili & cheese	1	610	510
sour cream & chives	1	230	460
TACO SALAD			
taco salad	1 serving	1,260	430
taco sauce	1 pkt	105	10

❏ FATS, OILS, & SHORTENINGS
See also BUTTER & MARGARINE SPREADS

	Portion	Sodium (mg)	Calories
shortening			
special for confectionery: fractionated palm	1 c	0	1,927
	1 T	0	120
all other	1 c	0	1,812–1,845
	1 T	0	113–115

	Portion	Sodium (mg)	Calories
Fats			
beef tallow	1 c	tr	1,849
	1 T	0	116
lard (pork)	1 c	tr	1,849
	1 T	0	116
Oils			
olive	1 c	tr	1,909
	1 T	0	119
peanut	1 c	tr	1,909
	1 T	tr	119
safflower			
soybean	1 c	tr	1,927
	1 T	0	120
sunflower			
linoleic (<60%)	1 c	tr	1,927
	1 T	tr	120

▪ BRAND NAME

	Portion	Sodium (mg)	Calories
Arrowhead Mills			
all oils	1 T	0	120
Mazola			
corn oil	1 T	0	120
No-Stick	2½-second spray	0	6
Planters			
peanut oil	1 T	0	120

❑ FISH *See* SEAFOOD & SEAFOOD PRODUCTS

❑ FLOURS & CORNMEALS
See also NUTS & NUT-BASED BUTTERS, FLOURS, MEALS, MILKS, PASTES, & POWDERS; SEEDS & SEED-BASED BUTTERS, FLOURS, & MEALS

	Portion	Sodium (mg)	Calories
arrowroot flour	1 T	4	29
barley flour	1 T	tr	28
	1 c	3	401
buckwheat flour			
dark	1 oz	tr	92
carob flour	1 c	36	185

	Portion	Sodium (mg)	Calories
corn flour	1 c	1	431
corn flour, sifted			
masa harina	⅓ c	3	137
masa trigo	⅓ c	294	149
cornmeal			
degermed, enriched			
dry	1 c	1	502
cooked	1 c	264	120
white, self-rising, dry	1 oz or ⅙ c	352	98
whole-ground, dry			
unbolted	1 c	1	433
bolted	1 c	1	442
manioc (casava) flour	3½ oz	5	320
potato flour	1 c	62	622
rice bran	1 oz	5	80
rice flour	1 c	13	479
rice polish	1 oz	2	101
rye flour			
dark	3½ oz	1	419
light	3½ oz	1	364
rye wheat flour	1 c	tr	400
soy flour *See* SOYBEANS & SOYBEAN PRODUCTS			
wheat & gluten flour	1 c	3	529
wheat flour, enriched			
all-purpose			
sifted	1 c	2	420
unsifted	1 c	3	499
bread, sifted	1 c	2	409
cake or pastry, sifted	1 c	2	350
self-rising, unsifted	1 c	1,349	440
whole-wheat & soy flour	3½ oz	297	365
whole-wheat flour, from hard wheats	1 c	4	400
whole-wheat flour, straight, soft	3½ oz	2	364

▪ BRAND NAME

Argo
Argo & Kingsford's cornstarch	1 T	tr	30

Arrowhead Mills
barley flour	2 oz	2	200
brown rice flour	2 oz	5	200
buckwheat flour	2 oz	0	190
corn flour, yellow	2 oz	1	210
cornmeal			
blue	2 oz	2	210
hi-lysine	2 oz	1	210
yellow	2 oz	1	210
Ezekiel flour	2 oz	2	200
garbanzo flour	2 oz	15	200

	Portion	Sodium (mg)	Calories
millet flour	2 oz	2	185
oat flour	2 oz	1	200
pastry flour	2 oz	2	180
rye flour	2 oz	1	190
triticale flour	2 oz	1	190
unbleached white flour	2 oz	1	200
vital wheat gluten	1 oz	1	100
whole-wheat flour	2 oz	2	200
Aunt Jemima			
CORNMEAL			
bolted white, mix	⅙ c	337	99
bolted yellow, mix	⅙ c	369	97
enriched white	3 T	1	101
enriched yellow	3 T	1	101
self-rising white	⅙ c	381	98
self-rising white enriched bolted	⅙ c	382	99
FLOUR			
enriched self-rising	¼ c	368	109
Fearn			
rice flour	½ c	0	270
Featherweight			
potato starch	1 c	51	620
rice flour	1 c	7	500
Heckers			
unbleached flour	about 1 c or 4 oz	0	380–400
whole-wheat flour	about 1 c or 4 oz	0	400
Quaker Oats			
masa harina de maiz	⅓ c	2	137
masa trigo	⅓ c	794	149

❑ **FRANKFURTERS** *See* PROCESSED MEAT & POULTRY PRODUCTS

❑ **FRUIT, FRESH & PROCESSED**
See also PICKLES, OLIVES, RELISHES, & CHUTNEYS; SNACKS

acerolas, raw	1 c	7	31
apples			
raw			
w/skin	1 fruit = 4.9 oz	1	81

	Portion	Sodium (mg)	Calories
w/out skin	1 fruit = 4½ oz	0	72
baked in microwave, w/out skin	½ c sliced	1	48
boiled, w/out skin	½ c sliced	1	46
canned, sweetened, unheated	½ c sliced	3	68
dehydrated, sulfured			
cooked	½ c	25	71
uncooked	½ c	37	104
dried, sulfured			
cooked, w/added sugar	½ c	27	116
cooked, w/out added sugar	½ c	26	72
uncooked	2¼ oz	56	155
	1 c	75	209
frozen, unsweetened			
heated	½ c sliced	3	48
unheated	½ c sliced	3	41
applesauce, canned			
sweetened	½ c	4	97
unsweetened	½ c	2	53
apricots			
raw	3 fruit = 3.7 oz	1	51
canned, w/skin			
in water	3 halves + 1¾ T liquid	2	22
in juice	3 halves + 1¾ T liquid	3	40
in extra-light syrup	3 halves + 1¾ T liquid	2	41
in light syrup	3 halves + 1¾ T liquid	3	54
in heavy syrup	3 halves + 1¾ T liquid	3	70
canned, w/out skin			
in water	2 fruit + 2 T liquid	10	20
in heavy syrup	2 fruit + 2 T liquid	9	75
in extra-heavy syrup	2 fruit + 2 T liquid	12	87
dehydrated (low-moisture), sulfured			
cooked	½ c	6	156
uncooked	½ c	8	192
dried, sulfured			
cooked, w/added sugar	½ c halves	4	153
cooked, w/out added sugar	½ c halves	4	106
uncooked	10 halves	3	83
frozen, sweetened	½ c	5	119

	Portion	Sodium (mg)	Calories
avocados, raw			
California	1 fruit = 6.1 oz	21	306
	1 c puree	28	407
Florida	1 fruit = 10.7 oz	14	339
	1 c puree	11	257
other commercial varieties	1 fruit = 7.1 oz	21	324
	1 c puree	24	370
bananas			
raw	1 fruit = 4 oz	1	105
dehydrated (banana powder)	1 T	0	21
blackberries			
raw	½ c	0	37
canned, in heavy syrup	½ c	3	118
frozen, unsweetened	1 c	2	97
blueberries			
raw	1 c	9	82
canned, in heavy syrup	½ c	4	112
frozen			
sweetened	1 c	3	187
unsweetened	1 c	1	78
boysenberries			
canned, in heavy syrup	½ c	4	113
frozen, unsweetened	1 c	2	66
breadfruit, raw	¼ small fruit = 3.4 oz	2	99
candied fruit *See* BAKING INGREDIENTS			
cantaloupe *See* melons, *below*			
carambolas, raw	1 fruit = 4½ oz	2	42
carissa plums, raw	1 fruit = 0.7 oz	1	12
casaba *See* melons, *below*			
cherries, sour, red			
raw	1 c w/pits	3	51
canned			
in water	½ c	9	43
in light syrup	½ c	9	94
in heavy syrup	½ c	9	116
in extra-heavy syrup	½ c	9	148
frozen, unsweetened	1 c	1	72
cherries, sweet			
raw	10 fruit = 2.4 oz	0	49
canned			
in water	½ c	2	57

	Portion	Sodium (mg)	Calories
in juice	½ c	3	68
in light syrup	½ c	3	85
in heavy syrup	½ c	3	107
in extra-heavy syrup	½ c	3	133
frozen, sweetened	1 c	3	232
Chinese gooseberries *See* kiwi fruit, *below*			
coconut *See* BAKING INGREDIENTS; NUTS & NUT-BASED BUTTERS, FLOURS, MEALS, MILKS, PASTES, & POWDERS			
crabapples, raw	1 c sliced	1	83
cranberries, raw	1 c whole	1	46
cranberry sauce, canned, sweetened	½ c	40	209
currants			
European, black, raw	½ c	1	36
red & white, raw	½ c	1	31
zante, dried	½ c	6	204
custard apples, raw	edible portion = 3½ oz	4	101
dates, domestic, dry	10 fruit = 2.9 oz	2	228
figs			
raw	1 medium fruit = 1¾ oz	1	37
canned			
in water	3 fruit + 1¾ T liquid	1	42
in light syrup	3 fruit + 1¾ T liquid	1	58
in heavy syrup	3 fruit + 1¾ T liquid	1	75
in extra-heavy syrup	3 fruit + 1¾ T liquid	1	91
dried			
cooked	½ c	6	140
uncooked	10 fruit = 6.6 oz	20	477
fruit cocktail, canned			
in water	½ c	5	40
in juice	½ c	4	56
in extra-light syrup	½ c	5	55
in light syrup	½ c	7	72
in heavy syrup	½ c	7	93
in extra-heavy syrup	½ c	7	115
fruit salad, canned			
in water	½ c	4	37
in juice	½ c	7	62
in light syrup	½ c	7	73
in heavy syrup	½ c	7	94
in extra-heavy syrup	½ c	7	114
fruit salad, tropical, canned, in heavy syrup	½ c	3	110

	Portion	Sodium (mg)	Calories
gooseberries			
raw	1 c	1	67
canned, in light syrup	½ c	3	93
grandillas *See* passion fruit, *below*			
grapefruit			
raw, pink & red	½ fruit = 4.3 oz	0	37
raw, white	½ fruit = 4.2 oz	0	39
canned			
in water	½ c	2	44
in juice	½ c	9	46
in light syrup	½ c	2	76
grapes			
American type, raw	10 fruit = 0.8 oz	0	15
European type, raw	10 fruit = 1.8 oz	1	36
Thompson seedless, canned			
in water	½ c	7	48
in heavy syrup, solids & liquids	½ c	7	94
guava sauce, cooked	½ c	4	43
guavas			
common, raw	1 fruit = 3.2 oz	2	45
strawberry, raw	1 fruit = 0.2 oz	2	4
honeydew *See* melons, *below*			
jackfruit, raw	edible portion = 3½ oz	3	94
jujubes			
raw	edible portion = 3½ oz	3	79
dried	edible portion = 3½ oz	9	287
kiwi fruit, raw	1 medium fruit = 2.7 oz	4	46
kumquats, raw	1 fruit = 0.7 oz	1	12
lemon peel, raw	1 T	0	
lemons, raw			
w/peel	1 medium fruit = 3.8 oz	3	22
w/out peel	1 medium fruit = 2 oz	1	17
limes, raw	1 fruit = 2.4 oz	1	20
litchis *See* lychees, *below*			
loganberries, frozen	1 c	1	80

	Portion	Sodium (mg)	Calories
longans			
raw	1 fruit = 0.1 oz	0	2
dried	edible portion = 3½ oz	48	286
loquats, raw	1 fruit = 0.3 oz	0	5
lychees			
raw	1 fruit = 0.3 oz	0	6
dried	edible portion = 3½ oz	3	277
mammy apples, raw	1 fruit = 29.8 oz	127	431
mangos, raw	1 fruit = 7.3 oz	4	135
melon balls, frozen, cantaloupe & honeydew	1 c	53	55
melons			
cantaloupe, raw	½ fruit = 9.4 oz	23	94
	1 c cubed	14	57
casaba, raw	⅒ fruit = 5.8 oz	20	43
	1 c cubed	20	45
honeydew, raw	⅒ fruit = 4½ oz	13	46
	1 c cubed	17	60
muskmelons *See* melons: cantaloupe, *above*			
mixed fruit			
canned, in heavy syrup, solids & liquids	½ c	5	92
dried	11 oz	52	712
frozen, sweetened	1 c	8	245
mulberries, raw	10 fruit = ½ oz	2	7
muskmelons *See* melons: cantaloupe, *above*			
natal plums *See* carissa plums, *above*			
nectarines, raw	1 fruit = 4.8 oz	0	67
oheloberries, raw	10 fruit = 0.4 oz	0	3
orange peel, raw	1 T	0	
oranges, raw			
w/peel	1 fruit = 5.6 oz	3	64
w/out peel			
California, navels	1 fruit = 4.9 oz	1	65
California, Valencias	1 fruit = 4.3 oz	0	59

	Portion	Sodium (mg)	Calories
oranges, raw: w/out peel *(cont.)*			
Florida	1 fruit = 5.3 oz	1	69
other commercial varieties	1 fruit = 4.6 oz	0	62
papayas, raw	1 fruit = 10.7 oz	8	117
passion fruit, purple, raw	1 fruit = 0.6 oz	5	18
peaches			
raw	1 fruit = 3.1 oz	0	37
canned, clingstone			
in water	1 half + 1⅔ T liquid	3	18
in extra-light syrup	1 half + 1⅔ T liquid	4	32
in light syrup	1 half + 1¾ T liquid	4	44
canned, clingstone & freestone			
in juice	1 half + 1⅔ T liquid	3	34
in heavy syrup	1 half + 1¾ T liquid	5	60
canned, freestone, in extra-heavy syrup	1 half + 1¾ T liquid	6	77
dehydrated (low-moisture), sulfured			
cooked	½ c	5	161
uncooked	½ c	6	188
dried, sulfured			
cooked, w/added sugar	½ c halves	3	139
cooked, w/out added sugar	½ c halves	3	99
uncooked	10 halves	9	311
frozen, sweetened	1 c sliced, thawed	16	235
peaches, spiced, canned, in heavy syrup	1 fruit + 2 T liquid	3	66
pears			
raw	1 fruit = 5.8 oz	1	98
canned			
in water	1 half + 1⅔ T liquid	2	22
in juice	1 half + 1⅔ T liquid	3	38
in extra-light syrup	1 half + 1⅔ T liquid	2	36
in light syrup	1 half + 1¾ T liquid	4	45

	Portion	Sodium (mg)	Calories
in heavy syrup	1 half + 1¾ T liquid	4	58
in extra-heavy syrup	1 half + 1¾ T liquid	4	77
dried, sulfured			
cooked, w/added sugar	½ c halves	4	196
cooked, w/out added sugar	½ c halves	4	163
uncooked	10 halves	10	459
persimmons			
Japanese			
raw	1 fruit = 5.9 oz	3	118
dried	1 fruit = 1.2 oz	1	93
native, raw	1 fruit = 0.9 oz	0	32
pineapple			
raw	1 slice = 3 oz	1	42
	1 c diced	1	77
canned			
in water	1 slice + 1¼ T liquid	1	19
	1 c tidbits	3	79
in juice	1 slice + 1¼ T liquid	1	35
	1 c chunks or tidbits	4	150
in light syrup	1 slice + 1¼ T liquid	1	30
	1 c	3	131
in heavy syrup	1 slice + 1¼ T liquid	1	45
	1 c chunks, tidbits, or crushed	3	199
in extra-heavy syrup	1 slice + 1¼ T liquid	1	48
	1 c chunks or crushed	3	217
frozen, sweetened	½ c chunks	2	104
pitangas, raw	1 fruit = 0.2 oz	0	2
	1 c	5	57
plantains			
raw	1 fruit = 6.3 oz	7	218
cooked	½ c sliced	4	89
plums, purple			
raw	1 fruit = 2.3 oz	0	36

	Portion	Sodium (mg)	Calories
plums, purple *(cont.)*			
canned			
in water	3 fruit + 2 T liquid	1	39
	1 c	2	102
in juice	3 fruit + 2 T liquid	1	55
	1 c	3	146
in light syrup	3 fruit + 2¾ T liquid	26	83
	1 c	50	158
in heavy syrup	3 fruit + 2¾ T liquid	26	119
	1 c	50	230
in extra-heavy syrup	3 fruit + 2¾ T liquid	25	135
	1 c	50	265
pomegranates, raw	1 fruit = 5.4 oz	5	104
prickly pears, raw	1 fruit = 3.6 oz	6	42
prunes			
canned, in heavy syrup	5 fruit + 2 T liquid	2	90
	1 c	6	245
dehydrated (low-moisture)			
cooked	½ c	3	158
uncooked	½ c	4	224
dried			
cooked, w/added sugar	½ c	2	147
cooked, w/out added sugar	½ c	2	113
uncooked	10 fruit = 3 oz	3	201
	1 c	6	385
pummelos, raw	1 fruit = 21.4 oz	7	228
	1 c sections	2	71
quinces, raw	1 fruit = 3.2 oz	4	53
raisins			
golden seedless	1 c not packed	17	437
	1 c packed	20	498
seeded	1 c not packed	41	428
	1 c packed	47	488
seedless	1 c not packed	17	434
	1 c packed	19	494
raspberries, red			
raw	1 c	0	61

	Portion	Sodium (mg)	Calories
canned, in heavy syrup, solids & liquids	½ c	4	117
frozen, sweetened	1 c	1	256
	10 oz pkg	1	291
rhubarb			
raw	½ c diced	2	13
frozen			
cooked, w/added sugar	½ c	2	139
uncooked	½ c	1	14
rose apples, raw	edible portion = 3½ oz	0	25
roselles, raw	1 c	3	28
sapodillas, raw	1 fruit = 6 oz	20	140
sapotes, raw	1 fruit = 7.9 oz	21	301
soursops, raw	1 fruit = 22 oz	87	416
startruit See carambolas, above			
strawberries			
raw	1 c	2	45
canned, in heavy syrup	½ c	5	117
frozen, sweetened			
whole	1 c	3	200
	10 oz pkg	3	223
sliced	1 c	8	245
	10 oz pkg	9	273
frozen, unsweetened	1 c	3	52
sugar apples, raw	1 fruit = 5½ oz	15	146
Surinam cherries See pitangas, above			
sweetsops See sugar apples, above			
tamarinds, raw	1 fruit = 0.1 oz	1	5
tangerines			
raw	1 fruit = 3 oz	1	37
canned			
in juice, solids & liquids	½ c	7	46
in light syrup, solids & liquids	½ c	8	76
watermelon, raw	1/16 fruit = 17 oz	10	152
	1 c diced	3	50
West Indian cherries See acerolas, above			

▪ BRAND NAME

Birds Eye

mixed fruit in syrup	5 oz	5	120
red raspberries in lite syrup	5 oz	0	100

	Portion	Sodium (mg)	Calories
strawberries, halved, in lite syrup	5 oz	5	90
strawberries, halved, in syrup	5 oz	0	120
Dole			
mandarin oranges in light syrup	½ c	8	76
pineapple cuts in juice	½ c	1	70
pineapple cuts in syrup	½ c	2	95
Dromedary			
chopped dates	¼ c	0	130
pitted dates	5	0	100
Fresh Chef			
Tropical Delight fruit salad	7 oz	270	240
Mott's			
applesauce	4 oz	<1	100
cinnamon applesauce	4 oz	<1	101
natural applesauce	4 oz	2	53
Mrs. Paul's			
apple fritters	2	610	270

❑ FRUIT & NUT SNACK MIXES
See SNACKS

❑ FRUIT CHUTNEYS & RELISHES
See PICKLES, OLIVES, RELISHES, & CHUTNEYS

❑ FRUIT SAUCES *See* FRUITS, FRESH & PROCESSED

❑ FRUIT SPREADS

Jams

average, all varieties, low-cal	1 T	16	29

Jellies

average, all varieties, low-cal	1 T	tr	27
blackberry	1 T	4	51
boysenberry	1 T	3	52
cherry	1 T	3	52
currant	1 T	8	52
grape	1 T	3	55

	Portion	Sodium (mg)	Calories
guava	1 T	3	52
quince	1 T	3	51
strawberry	1 T	2	51

Marmalades

citrus	1 T	3	51
orange	1 T	4	56

Preserves

apricot	1 T	2	51
apricot-pineapple	1 T	3	51
blackberry	1 T	2	55
boysenberry	1 T	6	54
peach	1 T	4	51

▪ BRAND NAME

Smucker's
FRUIT BUTTERS

apple	2 t	0	24
peach	2 t	0	30

JAMS, JELLIES, MARMALADES, & PRESERVES

all flavors			
regular	2 t	0	35
low-sugar	2 t	<10	16
Slenderella	2 t	0	32
imitation grape jelly or strawberry jam, artificially sweetened	2 t	3	4
orange marmalade	2 t	0	36

❏ GELATIN & GELATIN DESSERTS
See DESSERTS: CUSTARDS, GELATINS, PUDDINGS, & PIE FILLINGS

❏ GRAINS *See* RICE & GRAINS, PLAIN & PREPARED

❏ GRAVIES *See* SAUCES, GRAVIES, & CONDIMENTS

	Portion	Sodium (mg)	Calories

❑ **HAM** *See* PORK, FRESH & CURED;
PROCESSED MEAT & POULTRY PRODUCTS

❑ **HERBS & SPICES** *See* SEASONINGS

❑ **HONEY** *See* SUGARS & SWEETENERS

❑ **HOT DOGS** *See* frankfurters, *under*
PROCESSED MEAT & POULTRY PRODUCTS

❑ **ICE CREAM & ICE MILK**
See DESSERTS, FROZEN

❑ **INFANT & TODDLER FOODS**

Baked Products

	Portion	Sodium (mg)	Calories
arrowroot cookies	1	22	24
	1 oz	105	125
pretzels	1	16	24
	1 oz	76	113
teething biscuits	1	40	43
	1 oz	103	111
zwieback	1	16	30
	1 oz	66	121

Cereals, Hot & Cold

	Portion	Sodium (mg)	Calories
barley			
dry	½ oz	7	52
	1 T	1	9
w/whole milk	1 oz	14	31
cereal & egg yolks			
strained	about 4½ oz	42	66
	1 oz	9	15
junior	about 7½ oz	70	110
	1 oz	9	15
cereal, egg yolks, & bacon			
strained	about 4½ oz	62	101
	1 oz	14	22
junior	about 7½ oz	97	178
	1 oz	13	24
high protein			
dry	½ oz	7	51
	1 T	1	9

	Portion	Sodium (mg)	Calories
w/whole milk	1 oz	14	31
high protein w/apple & orange			
dry	½ oz	15	53
	1 T	2	9
w/whole milk	1 oz	16	32
mixed			
dry	½ oz	6	54
	1 T	1	9
w/whole milk	1 oz	13	32
mixed w/applesauce & bananas			
strained	about 4.8 oz	3	111
	1 oz	1	23
junior	about 7.8 oz	78	183
	1 oz	10	24
mixed w/bananas			
dry	½ oz	17	56
	1 T	3	9
w/whole milk	1 oz	17	33
mixed w/honey			
dry	½ oz	6	55
	1 T	1	9
w/whole milk	1 oz	14	33
oatmeal			
dry	½ oz	5	56
	1 T	1	10
w/whole milk	1 oz	13	33
oatmeal w/applesauce & bananas			
strained	about 4.8 oz	2	99
	1 oz	1	21
junior	about 7.8 oz	69	165
	1 oz	9	21
oatmeal w/bananas			
dry	½ oz	17	56
	1 T	3	9
w/whole milk	1 oz	17	33
oatmeal w/honey			
dry	½ oz	7	55
	1 T	1	9
w/whole milk	1 oz	14	33
rice			
dry	½ oz	5	56
	1 T	1	9
w/whole milk	1 oz	13	33
rice w/applesauce & bananas, strained	about 4.8 oz	38	107
	1 oz	8	23
rice w/bananas			
dry	½ oz	14	57
	1 T	2	10

	Portion	Sodium (mg)	Calories
rice w/bananas *(cont.)*			
w/whole milk	1 oz	16	33
rice w/honey			
dry	½ oz	7	56
	1 T	1	9
w/whole milk	1 oz	14	33
rice w/mixed fruit, junior	about 7.8 oz	24	186
	1 oz	3	24

Desserts

	Portion	Sodium (mg)	Calories
apple Betty			
strained	about 4.8 oz	14	97
	1 oz	3	20
junior	about 7.8 oz	19	153
	1 oz	2	20
caramel pudding			
strained	about 4.8 oz	37	104
	1 oz	8	22
junior	about 7½ oz	60	167
	1 oz	8	22
cherry vanilla pudding			
strained	about 4.8 oz	22	91
	1 oz	5	19
junior	about 7.8 oz	32	152
	1 oz	4	20
chocolate custard pudding			
strained	about 4½ oz	30	107
	1 oz	7	24
junior	about 7.8 oz	55	195
	1 oz	7	25
cottage cheese w/pineapple			
strained	about 4.8 oz	70	94
	1 oz	15	20
junior	about 7.8 oz	113	172
	1 oz	15	22
Dutch apple			
strained	about 4.8 oz	21	92
	1 oz	5	19
junior	about 7.8 oz	36	151
	1 oz	5	19
fruit dessert			
strained	about 4.8 oz	18	79
	1 oz	4	17
junior	about 7.8 oz	29	138
	1 oz	4	18
peach cobbler			
strained	about 4.8 oz	10	88
	1 oz	2	18
junior	about 7.8 oz	20	147
	1 oz	3	19

	Portion	Sodium (mg)	Calories
peach melba			
strained	about 4.8 oz	12	81
	1 oz	2	17
junior	about 7.8 oz	19	132
	1 oz	2	17
pineapple orange, strained	about 4½ oz	13	89
	1 oz	3	20
pineapple pudding			
strained	about 4½ oz	24	104
	1 oz	5	23
junior	about 7.8 oz	48	192
	1 oz	6	25
tropical fruit, junior	about 7.8 oz	16	131
	1 oz	2	17
vanilla custard pudding			
strained	about 4½ oz	36	109
	1 oz	8	24
junior	about 7.8 oz	64	196
	1 oz	8	25

Dinners, Regular

	Portion	Sodium (mg)	Calories
beef & egg noodles			
strained	about 4½ oz	37	68
	1 oz	8	15
junior	about 7½ oz	37	122
	1 oz	5	16
beef & rice, toddler	about 6.2 oz	632	146
	1 oz	101	23
beef lasagna, toddler	about 6.2 oz	804	137
	1 oz	129	22
beef stew, toddler	about 6.2 oz	611	90
	1 oz	98	14
chicken & noodles			
strained	about 4½ oz	20	67
	1 oz	5	15
junior	about 7½ oz	36	109
	1 oz	5	15
chicken soup, cream of, strained	about 4½ oz	24	74
	1 oz	5	16
chicken soup, strained	about 4½ oz	20	64
	1 oz	5	14
chicken stew, toddler	about 6 oz	683	132
	1 oz	114	22
lamb & noodles, junior	about 7.5 oz	39	138
	1 oz	5	18
macaroni & bacon, toddler	about 7½ oz	166	160
	1 oz	22	21

	Portion	Sodium (mg)	Calories
macaroni & cheese			
strained	about 4½ oz	93	76
	1 oz	13	17
junior	about 7½ oz	163	130
	1 oz	22	17
macaroni & ham, junior	about 7½ oz	101	127
	1 oz	13	17
macaroni, tomato, & beef			
strained	about 4½ oz	21	71
	1 oz	5	16
junior	about 7½ oz	35	125
	1 oz	5	17
mixed vegetables			
strained	about 4½ oz	10	52
	1 oz	2	11
junior	about 7½ oz	19	71
	1 oz	2	9
spaghetti, tomato, & meat			
junior	about 7½ oz	42	135
	1 oz	6	18
toddler	about 6.2 oz	634	133
	1 oz	101	21
split peas & ham, junior	about 7½ oz	30	152
	1 oz	4	20
turkey & rice			
strained	about 4½ oz	21	63
	1 oz	5	14
junior	about 7½ oz	33	104
	1 oz	4	14
vegetables & bacon			
strained	about 4½ oz	55	88
	1 oz	12	19
junior	about 7½ oz	96	150
	1 oz	13	20
vegetables & beef			
strained	about 4½ oz	27	67
	1 oz	6	15
junior	about 7½ oz	52	113
	1 oz	7	15
vegetables & chicken			
strained	about 4½ oz	14	55
	1 oz	3	12
junior	about 7½ oz	18	106
	1 oz	2	14
vegetables & ham			
strained	about 4½ oz	15	62
	1 oz	3	14
junior	about 7½ oz	37	110
	1 oz	5	15
toddler	about 6.2 oz	531	128
	1 oz	85	21

	Portion	Sodium (mg)	Calories
vegetables & lamb			
strained	about 4½ oz	26	67
	1 oz	6	15
junior	about 7½ oz	28	108
	1 oz	4	14
vegetables & liver			
strained	about 4½ oz	24	50
	1 oz	5	11
junior	about 7½ oz	27	93
	1 oz	4	12
vegetables & turkey			
strained	about 4½ oz	17	54
	1 oz	4	12
junior	about 7½ oz	36	101
	1 oz	5	13
toddler	about 6.2 oz	591	141
	1 oz	95	23
vegetables, dumplings, & beef			
strained	about 4½ oz	62	61
	1 oz	14	14
junior	about 7½ oz	110	103
	1 oz	15	14
vegetables, noodles, & chicken			
strained	about 4½ oz	26	81
	1 oz	6	18
junior	about 7½ oz	54	137
	1 oz	7	18
vegetables, noodles, & turkey			
strained	about 4½ oz	27	56
	1 oz	6	12
junior	about 7½ oz	37	110
	1 oz	5	15

Dinners, High in Meat or Cheese

	Portion	Sodium (mg)	Calories
beef w/vegetables			
strained	about 4½ oz	46	96
	1 oz	10	21
junior	about 4½ oz	42	108
	1 oz	9	24
chicken w/vegetables			
strained	about 4½ oz	35	100
	1 oz	8	22
junior	about 4½ oz	33	117
	1 oz	7	26
cottage cheese w/pineapple, strained	about 4.8 oz	201	157
	1 oz	42	33
ham w/vegetables			
strained	about 4½ oz	29	97
	1 oz	6	21

	Portion	Sodium (mg)	Calories
ham w/vegetables *(cont.)*			
junior	about 4½ oz	28	98
	1 oz	6	22
turkey w/vegetables			
strained	about 4½ oz	38	111
	1 oz	8	25
junior	about 4½ oz	56	115
	1 oz	12	25
veal w/vegetables			
strained	about 4½ oz	30	89
	1 oz	7	20
junior	about 4½ oz	32	93
	1 oz	7	21

Fruit
See also Desserts, *above*

	Portion	Sodium (mg)	Calories
apple blueberry			
strained	about 4.8 oz	2	82
	1 oz	0	17
junior	about 7.8 oz	28	137
	1 oz	4	18
apple raspberry			
strained	about 4.8 oz	3	79
	1 oz	1	17
junior	about 7.8 oz	4	127
	1 oz	0	16
applesauce			
strained	about 4½ oz	3	53
	1 oz	1	12
junior	about 7½ oz	5	79
	1 oz	1	11
applesauce & apricots			
strained	about 4.8 oz	4	60
	1 oz	1	13
junior	about 7.8 oz	6	104
	1 oz	1	13
applesauce & cherries			
strained	about 4.8 oz	3	65
	1 oz	1	14
junior	about 7.8 oz	6	106
	1 oz	1	14
applesauce & pineapple			
strained	about 4½ oz	3	48
	1 oz	1	11
junior	about 7½ oz	4	83
	1 oz	1	11
apricots w/tapioca			
strained	about 4.8 oz	11	80
	1 oz	2	17

	Portion	Sodium (mg)	Calories
junior	about 7.8 oz	14	139
	1 oz	2	18
bananas & pineapple w/tapioca			
strained	about 4.8 oz	10	91
	1 oz	2	19
junior	about 7.8 oz	13	143
	1 oz	2	18
bananas w/tapioca			
strained	about 4.8 oz	12	77
	1 oz	3	16
junior	about 7.8 oz	21	147
	1 oz	3	19
guava & papaya w/tapioca,	about 4½ oz	2	80
strained	1 oz	1	18
guava w/tapioca, strained	about 4½ oz	5	86
	1 oz	1	19
mango w/tapioca, strained	about 4.8 oz	6	109
	1 oz	1	23
papaya & applesauce w/tap-	about 4½ oz	6	89
ioca, strained	1 oz	1	20
peaches			
strained	about 4.8 oz	8	96
	1 oz	2	20
junior	about 7.8 oz	10	157
	1 oz	1	20
pears			
strained	about 4½ oz	3	53
	1 oz	1	12
junior	about 7½ oz	4	93
	1 oz	1	12
pears & pineapple			
strained	about 4½ oz	5	52
	1 oz	1	12
junior	about 7½ oz	2	93
	1 oz	0	12
plums w/tapioca			
strained	about 4.8 oz	8	96
	1 oz	2	20
junior	about 7.8 oz	18	163
	1 oz	2	21
prunes w/tapioca			
strained	about 4.8 oz	6	94
	1 oz	1	20
junior	about 7.8 oz	5	155
	1 oz	1	20

	Portion	Sodium (mg)	Calories
Fruit Juices			
apple	about 4.2 oz	4	61
	1 fl oz	1	14
apple-cherry	about 4.2 oz	4	53
	1 fl oz	1	13
apple-grape	about 4.2 oz	4	60
	1 fl oz	1	14
apple-prune	about 4.2 oz	7	94
	1 fl oz	2	23
mixed fruit	about 4.2 oz	5	61
	1 fl oz	1	14
orange	about 4.2 oz	2	58
	1 fl oz	0	14
orange-apple	about 4.2 oz	4	56
	1 fl oz	1	13
orange-apple-banana	about 4.2 oz	6	61
	1 fl oz	1	15
orange-apricot	about 4.2 oz	7	60
	1 fl oz	2	14
orange-banana	about 4.2 oz	4	65
	1 fl oz	1	15
orange-pineapple	about 4.2 oz	2	63
	1 fl oz	1	15
prune-orange	about 4.2 oz	2	91
	1 fl oz	1	22
Meats & Egg Yolks			
beef			
strained	about 3½ oz	80	106
	1 oz	23	30
junior	about 3½ oz	65	105
	1 oz	19	30
beef w/beef heart, strained	about 3½ oz	62	93
	1 oz	18	27
chicken			
strained	about 3½ oz	47	128
	1 oz	13	37
junior	about 3½ oz	50	148
	1 oz	14	42
chicken sticks, junior	1 stick = 0.35 oz	48	19
	2½ oz	340	134
egg yolks, strained	about 3.3 oz	37	191
	1 oz	11	58
ham			
strained	about 3½ oz	40	110
	1 oz	12	32
junior	about 3½ oz	66	123
	1 oz	19	35

	Portion	Sodium (mg)	Calories
lamb			
strained	about 3½ oz	62	102
	1 oz	18	29
junior	about 3½ oz	73	111
	1 oz	21	32
liver, strained	about 3½ oz	73	100
	1 oz	21	29
meat sticks, junior	1 stick = 0.35 oz	55	18
	2½ oz	388	130
pork, strained	about 3½ oz	42	123
	1 oz	12	35
turkey			
strained	about 3½ oz	54	113
	1 oz	16	32
junior	about 3½ oz	72	128
	1 oz	20	37
turkey sticks, junior	1 stick = 0.35 oz	48	18
	2½ oz	343	129
veal			
strained	about 3½ oz	64	100
	1 oz	18	29
junior	about 3½ oz	68	109
	1 oz	19	31

Vegetables

	Portion	Sodium (mg)	Calories
beans, green			
plain			
strained	about 4½ oz	2	32
	1 oz	1	7
junior	about 7.3 oz	3	51
	1 oz	0	7
buttered			
strained	about 4½ oz	4	42
	1 oz	1	9
junior	about 7.3 oz	4	67
	1 oz	1	9
creamed, junior	about 7½ oz	26	68
	1 oz	3	9
beets, strained	about 4½ oz	106	43
	1 oz	24	10
carrots			
plain			
strained	about 4½ oz	48	34
	1 oz	11	8
junior	about 7½ oz	104	67
	1 oz	14	9

	Portion	Sodium (mg)	Calories
carrots *(cont.)*			
buttered			
strained	about 4½ oz	24	46
	1 oz	5	10
junior	about 7½ oz	34	70
	1 oz	5	9
corn, creamed			
strained	about 4½ oz	55	73
	1 oz	12	16
junior	about 7½ oz	111	138
	1 oz	15	18
garden vegetables, strained	about 4½ oz	45	48
	1 oz	10	11
mixed vegetables			
strained	about 4½ oz	16	52
	1 oz	4	11
junior	about 7½ oz	77	88
	1 oz	10	12
peas			
plain, strained	about 4½ oz	5	52
	1 oz	1	11
buttered			
strained	about 4½ oz	10	72
	1 oz	2	16
junior	about 7.3 oz	11	123
	1 oz	2	17
creamed, strained	about 4½ oz	18	68
	1 oz	4	15
spinach, creamed			
strained	about 4½ oz	62	48
	1 oz	14	11
junior	about 7½ oz	117	90
	1 oz	16	12
squash			
plain			
strained	about 4½ oz	229	30
	1 oz	51	7
junior	about 7½ oz	3	51
	1 oz	0	7
buttered			
strained	about 4½ oz	2	37
	1 oz	0	8
junior	about 7½ oz	3	63
	1 oz	0	8
sweet potatoes			
plain			
strained	about 4.8 oz	27	77
	1 oz	6	16
junior	about 7.8 oz	49	133
	1 oz	6	17

	Portion	Sodium (mg)	Calories
buttered			
strained	about 4.8 oz	11	76
	1 oz	2	16
junior	about 7.8 oz	17	126
	1 oz	2	16

▪ BRAND NAME

Beech-Nut
STAGE 1

Cereal

barley (calcium-fortified)	½ oz dry	20	50
	½ oz dry + 2.4 fl oz formula	40	100
oatmeal (calcium-fortified)	½ oz dry	15	50
	½ oz dry + 2.4 fl oz formula	35	100
rice (calcium-fortified)	½ oz dry	15	60
	½ oz dry + 2.4 fl oz formula	35	100

Fruit Juices

apple	4.2 fl oz	5	60
pear	4.2 fl oz	5	60
white grape	4.2 fl oz	10	80

Meat

beef	2.8 oz	40	90
chicken	2.8 oz	55	80
lamb	2.8 oz	50	70
turkey	2.8 oz	50	100
veal	2.8 oz	45	100

Vegetables

regal imperial carrots	4½ oz	130	40
sweet potatoes	4½ oz	60	70

STAGE 2

Cereals

mixed (calcium-fortified)	½ oz dry	15	50
	½ oz dry + 2.4 fl oz milk	50	100
w/applesauce & bananas	4½ oz	5	80

	Portion	Sodium (mg)	Calories
oatmeal			
w/applesauce & bananas	4½ oz	5	90
w/bananas (calcium-fortified)	½ oz dry	15	50
	½ oz dry + 2.4 fl oz milk	50	90
rice			
w/apples	½ oz dry	15	60
	½ oz dry + 2.4 fl oz milk	50	110
w/applesauce & bananas	4½ oz	25	100
w/bananas (calcium-fortified)	½ oz dry	15	60
Desserts			
banana custard	4½ oz	30	120
banana pineapple	4½ oz	15	100
Dutch apple	4½ oz	20	80
guava tropical fruit	4½ oz	10	100
mango tropical fruit	4½ oz	15	90
papaya tropical fruit	4½ oz	15	80
vanilla custard	4½ oz	16	130
Fruit & Dairy			
cottage cheese w/pineapple	4½ oz	15	110
mixed fruit & yogurt	4½ oz	20	110
peaches & yogurt	4½ oz	25	110
Fruit & Fruit Dishes			
apples, mandarin oranges, & bananas	4½ oz	5	90
applesauce & apricots	4½ oz	5	70
applesauce & bananas	4½ oz	5	70
applesauce & cherries	4½ oz	5	70
bartlett pears & pineapple	4½ oz	5	80
plums w/rice	4½ oz	10	110
Juice			
Juice Plus	4 fl oz	20	80
Main Courses			
beef & egg noodles w/vegetables	4½ oz	30	90
Beef Dinner Supreme	4½ oz	40	120
chicken & rice dinner	4½ oz	40	80
chicken noodle dinner	4½ oz	55	90
macaroni, tomato, & beef	4½ oz	40	90
Turkey Dinner Supreme	4½ oz	25	110
turkey rice dinner	4½ oz	35	70
vegetable beef	4½ oz	35	90
vegetable chicken	4½ oz	65	90
vegetable ham	4½ oz	30	90
vegetable lamb	4½ oz	40	90

	Portion	Sodium (mg)	Calories
Vegetables			
creamed corn	4½ oz	25	90
garden vegetables	4½ oz	25	60
mixed vegetables	4½ oz	30	50
peas & carrots	4½ oz	50	60
STAGE 3			
Custard			
vanilla	6 oz	70	120
Fruit & Dairy			
cottage cheese w/pineapple	6 oz	20	160
mixed fruit & yogurt	6 oz	30	140
Fruit & Fruit Dishes			
bartlett pears	6 oz	5	90
Main Courses & Dinners			
beef & egg noodles dinner	6 oz	45	180
chicken noodles dinner	6 oz	55	100
macaroni, tomato, & beef	6 oz	85	150
spaghetti, tomato, & beef	6 oz	75	150
turkey rice dinner	6 oz	65	110
vegetable beef	6 oz	70	160
vegetable chicken	6 oz	70	90
Vegetables			
carrots	6 oz	170	50
sweet potatoes	6 oz	80	90
UNSTAGED			
Juices			
apple	4 or 4.2 fl oz	5	60
apple cherry	4 or 4.2 fl oz	5	50
apple cranberry	4.2 fl oz	5	60
apple grape	4 or 4.2 fl oz	5	60
mixed fruit	4 or 4.2 fl oz	5	60
orange	4.2 fl oz	5	60
pear	4 or 4.2 fl oz	5	60
tropical blend	4 fl oz	10	70
TABLE TIME			
Main Courses			
beef stew	6 oz	300	150
spaghetti rings in meat sauce	6 oz	350	160
vegetable stew w/chicken	6 oz	300	190
Soups			
Hearty chicken w/stars	6 oz	300	180

	Portion	Sodium (mg)	Calories
Gerber			
BAKED GOODS			
animal crackers	4	46	50
animal-shaped cookies	2	19	60
arrowroot cookies	2	36	50
pretzels	2	59	50
Toddler Biter biscuits	1	29	50
zwieback toast	2	29	70
CHUNKY PRODUCTS			
Homestyle noodles & beef	6 oz	368	150
macaroni alphabets w/beef & tomato sauce	6¼ oz	354	140
noodles & chicken w/carrots & peas	6 oz	355	110
rice w/beef & tomato sauce	6¼ oz	361	140
saucy rice w/chicken	6 oz	381	120
spaghetti tomato sauce & beef	6¼ oz	398	160
vegetables & beef	6¼ oz	354	130
vegetables & chicken	6¼ oz	354	140
vegetables & ham	6¼ oz	373	130
vegetables & turkey	6¼ oz	366	120
DRY CEREALS, READY-TO-SERVE			
barley	½ oz dry	2	60
	½ oz dry + 2.4 fl oz milk	38	100
high protein	½ oz dry	1	50
	½ oz dry + 2.4 fl oz milk	37	100
w/apple & orange	½ oz dry	11	60
	½ oz dry + 2.4 fl oz milk	47	100
mixed	½ oz dry	1	50
	½ oz dry + 2.4 fl oz milk	37	100
w/banana	½ oz dry	13	60
	½ oz dry + 2.4 fl oz milk	49	100
oatmeal	½ oz dry	1	60
	½ oz dry + 2.4 fl oz milk	37	100
w/banana	½ oz dry	14	60
	½ oz dry + 2.4 fl oz milk	50	100
rice	½ oz dry	1	60
	½ oz dry + 2.4 fl oz milk	37	100

	Portion	Sodium (mg)	Calories
w/banana	½ oz dry	11	60
	½ oz dry + 2.4 fl oz milk	47	100

STRAINED FOODS

Cereals w/Fruit

mixed w/applesauce & bananas	4½ oz	4	100
oatmeal w/applesauce & bananas	4½ oz	4	100
rice w/applesauce & bananas	4½ oz	14	100

Desserts

banana apple	4½ oz	9	90
cherry vanilla pudding	4½ oz	12	90
chocolate custard pudding	4½ oz	29	110
Dutch apple	4½ oz	18	100
fruit	4½ oz	13	100
Hawaiian Delight	4½ oz	23	120
orange pudding	4½ oz	28	110
peach cobbler	4½ oz	9	100
vanilla custard pudding	4½ oz	32	100

Dinners, Regular

beef egg noodle	4½ oz	14	90
chicken noodle	4½ oz	17	90
macaroni cheese	4½ oz	108	90
macaroni tomato beef	4½ oz	41	80
turkey rice	4½ oz	20	80
vegetable bacon	4½ oz	68	100
vegetable beef	4½ oz	17	90
vegetable chicken	4½ oz	12	80
vegetable ham	4½ oz	14	80
vegetable lamb	4½ oz	17	90
vegetable liver	4½ oz	18	60
vegetable turkey	4½ oz	17	70

Dinners, Lean Meat

beef w/vegetables	4½ oz	32	90
chicken w/vegetables	4½ oz	31	90
ham w/vegetables	4½ oz	26	100
turkey w/vegetables	4½ oz	31	100

Fruit & Tropical Fruit

apple blueberry	4½ oz	1	60
applesauce	4½ oz	3	60
applesauce apricot	4½ oz	3	70
apricots w/tapioca	4½ oz	7	90
bananas w/pineapple & tapioca	4½ oz	5	60
bananas w/tapioca	4½ oz	12	110
guava w/tapioca	4½ oz	3	90

	Portion	Sodium (mg)	Calories
mango w/tapioca	4½ oz	4	90
papaya w/tapioca	4½ oz	9	80
peaches	4½ oz	4	90
pear pineapple	4½ oz	3	80
pears	4½ oz	3	80
plums w/tapioca	4½ oz	5	90
prunes w/tapioca	4½ oz	5	100
Juices			
apple	4.2 oz	3	60
apple apricot	4.2 oz	4	60
apple banana	4.2 oz	4	70
apple cherry	4.2 oz	5	60
apple grape	4.2 oz	5	60
apple peach	4.2 oz	5	60
apple pineapple	4.2 oz	3	60
apple plum	4.2 oz	7	60
apple prune	4.2 oz	5	70
mixed fruit	4.2 oz	3	70
orange	4.2 oz	5	70
pear	4.2 oz	7	60
Meats & Egg Yolks			
beef	2½ oz	38	80
chicken	2½ oz	28	110
egg yolks	2¼ oz	27	130
ham	2½ oz	30	90
lamb	2½ oz	36	70
pork	2½ oz	29	90
turkey	2½ oz	38	100
veal	2½ oz	38	80
Vegetables			
beets	4½ oz	115	60
carrots	4½ oz	46	40
creamed corn	4½ oz	12	80
creamed spinach	4½ oz	73	60
garden vegetables	4½ oz	26	50
green beans	4½ oz	1	50
mixed vegetables	4½ oz	15	60
peas	4½ oz	6	60
squash	4½ oz	3	40
sweet potatoes	4½ oz	22	80
FIRST FOODS			
Fruit			
applesauce	2½ oz	1	40
bananas	2½ oz	3	60

	Portion	Sodium (mg)	Calories
peaches	2½ oz	3	30
pears	2½ oz	2	40
prunes	2½ oz	4	70
Vegetables			
carrots	2½ oz	19	40
green beans	2½ oz	1	20
peas	2½ oz	2	40
squash	2½ oz	2	20
sweet potatoes	2½ oz	11	50
JUNIOR FOODS			
Cereals w/Fruit			
mixed w/applesauce & bananas	6 oz	5	140
oatmeal w/applesauce & bananas	6 oz	7	130
rice w/mixed fruit	6 oz	17	140
Desserts			
Dutch apple	6 oz	24	130
fruit	6 oz	12	130
Hawaiian Delight	6 oz	32	150
peach cobbler	6 oz	15	130
vanilla custard pudding	6 oz	41	150
Dinners, Regular			
beef egg noodle	6 oz	27	120
chicken noodle	6 oz	20	100
macaroni tomato beef	6 oz	27	110
spaghetti tomato sauce beef	6 oz	41	120
split peas ham	6 oz	27	130
turkey rice	6 oz	34	110
vegetable bacon	6 oz	105	140
vegetable beef	6 oz	31	110
vegetable chicken	6 oz	20	100
vegetable ham	6 oz	24	120
vegetable lamb	6 oz	29	120
vegetable turkey	6 oz	24	100
Dinners, Lean Meat			
beef w/vegetables	4½ oz	29	100
chicken w/vegetables	4½ oz	32	90
ham w/vegetables	4½ oz	27	110
turkey w/vegetables	4½ oz	31	100

	Portion	Sodium (mg)	Calories
Fruit			
apple blueberry	6 oz	2	80
applesauce	6 oz	3	90
apricots w/tapioca	6 oz	9	130
bananas w/pineapple & tapioca	6 oz	7	90
bananas w/tapioca	6 oz	15	140
peaches	6 oz	5	110
pear pineapple	6 oz	3	100
pears	6 oz	2	100
plums w/tapioca	6 oz	3	130
Meats			
beef	2½ oz	38	80
chicken	2½ oz	28	110
ham	2½ oz	30	90
turkey	2½ oz	37	100
veal	2½ oz	39	80
Vegetables			
carrots	6 oz	83	50
creamed green beans	6 oz	14	80
mixed vegetables	6 oz	32	70
peas	6 oz	5	90
squash	6 oz	3	60
sweet potatoes	6 oz	39	110
TODDLER FOODS			
Cereals			
Toasted Oat Rings	½ oz dry	33	60
	½ oz dry + 2.7 fl oz milk	74	110
Juices			
apple	4 oz	3	60
apple & berry	4 oz	8	60
apple cherry	4 oz	6	60
apple grape	4 oz	5	60
Fruits of the Sun	4 oz	4	60
Fruits-A-Plenty	4 oz	4	60
mixed fruit	4 oz	5	60
pear	4 oz	6	60
Meat & Poultry Sticks			
chicken	2½ oz	322	120
meat	2½ oz	329	110
turkey	2½ oz	307	120

	Portion	Sodium (mg)	Calories
Health Valley			
brown rice cereal	½ oz or 2 T	10	110
sprouted cereal	½ oz or 2 T	10	110
Nabisco			
zwieback teething toast	2	20	60

◻ **JAMS & JELLIES** *See* FRUIT SPREADS

◻ **JUICE, FROZEN** *See* DESSERTS, FROZEN

◻ **JUICES & JUICE DRINKS**
   See BEVERAGES

◻ **LAMB, VEAL,
   & MISCELLANEOUS MEATS**

Lamb, Cooked

	Portion	Sodium (mg)	Calories
lamb chops (3/lb w/bone)			
lean & fat			
arm, braised	2.2 oz	46	220
loin, broiled	2.8 oz	62	235
rib	3½ oz	83	423
lean only			
arm, braised	1.7 oz	36	135
loin, broiled	2.3 oz	54	140
leg of lamb, roasted			
lean & fat	3 oz	57	205
lean only	2.6 oz	50	140
rib, roasted			
lean & fat	3 oz	60	315
lean only	2 oz	46	130

Veal, Cooked

	Portion	Sodium (mg)	Calories
arm steak, lean & fat	3½ oz	51	298
blade, lean & fat	3½ oz	55	276
breast, stewed w/gravy	2.6 oz	64	256
cutlet, medium fat, bone removed			
braised or broiled	3 oz	56	185
breaded	3½ oz	54	319

	Portion	Sodium (mg)	Calories
flank, medium fat, stewed	3½ oz	80	390
foreshank, medium fat, stewed	3½ oz	80	216
loin chop, lean & fat	3½ oz	44	421
plate, medium fat, stewed	3½ oz	80	303
rib, roasted	3 oz	57	230

Other Meats

rabbit, stewed	3½ oz	41	216
venison, roasted	3½ oz	70	146
whale meat, raw	3½ oz	78	156

❑ LEGUMES & LEGUME PRODUCTS

Beans

adzuki			
boiled	½ c	9	147
canned, sweetened	½ c	323	351
yokan (sugar & bean confection)	1½ oz	12	36
black turtle soup			
boiled	1 c	6	241
canned	½ c	461	109
black, boiled	½ c	1	113
broad			
raw	½ c	9	256
boiled	½ c	4	93
canned, solids & liquids	½ c	580	91
cannellini *See* kidney, *below*			
cranberry			
boiled	½ c	1	120
canned, solids & liquids	½ c	431	108
fava *See* broad, *above*			
French, boiled	½ c	5	111
garbanzo *See* chickpeas, *under* Peas & Lentils, *below*			
great northern			
boiled	½ c	2	104
canned, solids & liquids	½ c	6	150
green gram *See* mung, *below*			
hyacinth, boiled	½ c	7	114
kidney			
California red, boiled	½ c	4	109
red			
boiled	½ c	2	112
canned, solids & liquids	½ c	437	108
royal red, boiled	½ c	4	108
other types			
boiled	½ c	2	112

	Portion	Sodium (mg)	Calories
canned, solids & liquids	½ c	445	104
lima			
baby			
boiled	½ c	2	115
frozen, boiled, drained	10 oz pkg	90	326
	½ c	26	94
large			
boiled	½ c	2	108
canned, solids & liquids	½ c	403	95
frozen, boiled, drained	10 oz pkg	164	312
	½ c	45	85
long rice *See* mung, *below*			
lupins, boiled	½ c	3	98
miso *See* fermented products, *under* SOYBEANS & SOYBEAN PRODUCTS			
moth, boiled	½ c	8	103
mung			
boiled	½ c	2	107
long rice, dehydrated, pre-pared from mung bean starch	½ c	7	246
mature seeds, sprouted			
raw	12 oz pkg	19	102
	½ c	3	16
boiled, drained	½ c	6	13
mungo, boiled	½ c	7	95
natto *See* fermented products, *under* SOYBEANS & SOYBEAN PRODUCTS			
navy, canned, solids & liquids	½ c	587	148
okara *See* tofu: okara, *under* SOYBEANS & SOYBEAN PRODUCTS			
pink, boiled	½ c	2	125
pinto			
boiled	½ c	1	117
canned, solids & liquids	½ c	499	93
Roman *See* cranberry, *above*			
shellie *See* beans, shellie, *under* VEGETABLES, PLAIN & PREPARED			
small white, boiled	½ c	2	127
snap *See* beans, snap, *under* VEGETABLES, PLAIN & PREPARED			
soybeans *See* SOYBEANS & SOYBEAN PRODUCTS			
tempeh *See* fermented products, *under* SOYBEANS & SOYBEAN PRODUCTS			
white			
boiled	½ c	6	125
canned, solids & liquids	½ c	7	153
winged			
raw	½ c	35	372
boiled	½ c	11	126
yardlong			
raw	½ c	14	292
boiled	½ c	4	102
yellow, boiled	½ c	4	126
yokan *See* adzuki, *above*			

	Portion	Sodium (mg)	Calories

Peas & Lentils

Bengal gram *See* chickpeas, *below*
black-eyed peas *See* cowpeas, common, *below*

chickpeas			
boiled	½ c	6	134
canned, solids & liquids	½ c	359	143
cowpeas, catjang, boiled	½ c	16	100
cowpeas, common			
boiled	½ c	3	100
canned, plain, solids & liquids	½ c	359	92
frozen, boiled, drained	½ c	5	112
cowpeas, leafy tips			
raw	1 c	2	10
boiled, drained	½ c	2	6
cowpeas, young pods w/seeds			
raw	1 pod = 0.4 oz	0	5
boiled, drained	½ c	1	16

crowder peas *See* cowpeas, common, *above*
golden gram *See* chickpeas, *above*

lentils			
boiled	½ c	2	115
sprouted, raw	½ c	4	40
pigeon peas			
raw	½ c	17	350
boiled	½ c	5	102

red gram *See* pigeon peas, *above*
southern peas *See* cowpeas, common, *above*

split peas, boiled	½ c	2	116

Prepared Bean Dishes

baked beans			
canned			
plain or vegetarian	½ c	504	118
w/franks	½ c	551	182
w/beef	½ c	632	161
w/pork	½ c	522	133
w/pork & tomato sauce	½ c	554	123
w/pork & sweet sauce	½ c	423	140
homemade	½ c	532	190
chili w/beans, canned	½ c	668	144
cowpeas, common, canned, w/ pork	½ c	420	99
falafel	0.6 oz	50	57
	1.8 oz	150	170
hummus	1 c	599	420
refried beans, canned	½ c	534	134

	Portion	Sodium (mg)	Calories

- **BRAND NAME**

Armour Star
chili
w/beans	7½ oz	1,190	390
w/out beans	7½ oz	1,150	390
Texas chili w/beans	7½ oz	1,270	370

Arrowhead Mills
adzuki beans	2 oz	5	190
anasazi beans	2 oz	6	200
black turtle beans	2 oz	15	190
chickpeas	2 oz	15	200
kidney beans	2 oz	5	190
lentils			
green	2 oz	15	190
red	2 oz	17	195
mung beans, sprouted	1 c	4	50
pinto beans	2 oz	5	200
split peas, green	2 oz	25	200

Campbell
barbecue beans	7⅞ oz	900	210
Home Style beans	8 oz	900	230
Old Fashioned beans in molasses & brown sugar	8 oz	730	230
pork & beans in tomato sauce	8 oz	730	190
Ranchero beans	7¾ oz	860	180

Fearn
BEAN MIXES
bean barley stew	½ of 3½ oz box	55	180
black bean Creole	½ of 3¾ oz box	20	180
lentil minestrone soup	½ of 3¾ oz box	825	160
split pea soup	½ of 3½ oz box	50	180
tri-bean casserole	½ of 3¼ oz box	15	160

VEGETARIAN MIXES
breakfast patty	⅛ of 7.4 oz box	250	110
falafel	⅑ of 7.4 oz box	250	80
sesame burger	¼ c dry or ⅛ of 8.4 oz box	100	130
sunflower burger	¼ c dry or ⅛ of 8.4 oz box	4	120

	Portion	Sodium (mg)	Calories
Featherweight			
chili w/beans	7½ oz	405	210
Health Valley			
BEANS			
Boston baked			
regular	4 oz	390	125
no salt	4 oz	25	125
vegetarian, w/miso	4 oz	310	110
CHILI			
con carne	4 oz	482	155
mild vegetarian w/beans			
regular	4 oz	430	145
no salt	4 oz	25	145
spicy vegetarian w/beans			
regular	4 oz	430	145
no salt	4 oz	25	145
w/lentils			
regular	4 oz	200	130
low-sodium	4 oz	50	142
LENTILS			
Zesty pilaf			
regular	4 oz	380	127
no salt	4 oz	15	127
Joan of Arc Canned Vegetables			
blackeye peas	½ c	300	90
butter beans	½ c	420	80
Caliente Style chili beans	½ c	620	100
garbanzo beans	½ c	320	90
great northern beans	½ c	290	80
kidney beans			
dark red	½ c	250	90
light red	½ c	250	90
pinto beans	½ c	280	90
pork & beans in tomato sauce	½ c	420	90
Van Camp's			
Beanee Weenee	1 c	990	326
brown sugar beans	1 c	692	284
butter beans	1 c	752	162
chili			
w/beans	1 c	1,215	352
w/out beans	1 c	1,499	412
kidney beans			
dark red	1 c	732	182
light red	1 c	688	184
New Orleans–style red	1 c	793	178

	Portion	Sodium (mg)	Calories
Mexican-style chili beans	1 c	718	210
pork & beans	1 c	1,011	216
red beans	1 c	928	194
vegetarian-style beans	1 c	987	206
Western-style beans	1 c	1,006	207
Wolf			
chili			
w/beans	1 c	1,013	345
w/out beans			
regular	1 c	1,042	387
extra spicy	scant c	962	363

❑ **LUNCHEON MEATS** *See* PROCESSED MEAT & POULTRY PRODUCTS

❑ **MAIN COURSES** *See* ENTREES & MAIN COURSES, CANNED & BOXED; ENTREES & MAIN COURSES, FROZEN

❑ **MARGARINE** *See* BUTTER & MARGARINE SPREADS

❑ **MARMALADE** *See* FRUIT SPREADS

❑ **MAYONNAISE** *See* SALAD DRESSINGS, MAYONNAISE, VINEGAR, & DIPS

❑ **MEAT** *See* BEEF, FRESH & CURED; LAMB, VEAL, & MISCELLANEOUS MEATS; PORK, FRESH & CURED; PROCESSED MEAT & POULTRY PRODUCTS

❑ **MEAT PRODUCTS, SIMULATED** *See* LEGUMES & LEGUME PRODUCTS; NUTS & NUT-BASED BUTTERS, FLOURS, MEALS, MILKS, PASTES, & POWDERS; SOYBEANS & SOYBEAN PRODUCTS

	Portion	Sodium (mg)	Calories

❏ **MEAT SPREADS** *See* PROCESSED MEAT & POULTRY PRODUCTS

❏ **MILK, MILK SUBSTITUTES, & MILK PRODUCTS: CREAM, SOUR CREAM, CREAM SUBSTITUTES, MILK, MILK SUBSTITUTES, WHEY, & YOGURT**

Cream & Sour Cream

CREAM

	Portion	Sodium (mg)	Calories
half & half	1 T	6	20
	1 c	98	315
light	1 T	6	29
	1 c	95	469
medium (25% fat)	1 T	6	37
	1 c	88	583
whipping			
light	1 T	5	44
	1 c or about 2 c whipped	82	699
heavy	1 T	6	52
	1 c or about 2 c whipped	89	821

SOUR CREAM

	Portion	Sodium (mg)	Calories
cultured	1 T	6	26
	1 c	123	493
half & half, cultured	1 T	6	20

Cream & Sour Cream Substitutes

	Portion	Sodium (mg)	Calories
coffee whitener, nondairy			
liquid, frozen, containing hydrogenated vegetable oil & soy protein	½ fl oz ½ c	12 95	20 163
liquid, frozen, containing lauric acid oil & sodium caseinate	½ fl oz ½ c	12 95	20 164
powdered, containing lauric acid oil & sodium caseinate	1 t	4	11
imitation sour cream, nondairy, cultured, containing lauric acid oil & sodium caseinate	1 oz 1 c	29 235	59 479

	Portion	Sodium (mg)	Calories
sour dressing, nonbutterfat,	1 T	6	21
cultured (made by combining fats or oils other than milk fat w/milk solids)	1 c	113	417

Milk, Cows'

FRESH

whole			
3.7% fat, pasteurized or raw	1 c	119	157
low-sodium	1 c	6	149
low-fat			
2% fat	1 c	122	121
2% fat, nonfat milk solids added	1 c	128	125
2% fat, protein-fortified	1 c	145	137
1% fat	1 c	123	102
1% fat, nonfat milk solids added	1 c	128	104
1% fat, protein-fortified	1 c	143	119
skim	1 c	126	86
skim, nonfat milk solids added	1 c	130	90
skim, protein-fortified	1 c	144	100
buttermilk, cultured	1 c	257	99

CONDENSED & EVAPORATED

condensed, sweetened, canned	1 oz	49	123
	1 c	389	982
evaporated, canned			
whole	1 oz	33	42
	½ c	133	169
skim	1 fl oz	37	25
	½ c	147	99

DRY

whole	¼ c	119	159
	1 c	475	635
nonfat			
regular	¼ c	161	109
	1 c	642	435
calcium-reduced	1 oz	646	100
instant	3.2 oz	499	326
	1 c	373	244
buttermilk, sweet cream	1 T	34	25
	1 c	621	464

	Portion	Sodium (mg)	Calories
Milk, Other			
goat	1 c	122	168
human	1 oz	5	21
Indian buffalo	1 c	127	236
sheep	1 c	108	264
Milk Substitutes			
filled (made by blending hydrogenated vegetable oils w/milk solids)	1 c	138	154
filled, w/lauric acid oil (made by combining milk solids w/fats or oils other than milk fat)	1 c	138	153
imitation, containing blend of hydrogenated vegetable oils	1 c	191	150
imitation, containing lauric acid	1 c	191	150
Whey			
acid			
dry	1 T	28	10
fluid	1 c	118	59
sweet			
dry	1 T	80	26
fluid	1 c	132	66
Yogurt			
coffee & vanilla varieties, low-fat, 11 g protein	1 c	149	194
fruit varieties, low-fat			
9 g protein	1 c	121	225
10 g protein	1 c	133	231
11 g protein	1 c	147	239
plain			
8 g protein	1 c	105	139
low-fat, 12 g protein	1 c	159	144
skim milk, 13 g protein	1 c	174	127

▪ BRAND NAME

	Portion	Sodium (mg)	Calories
Colombo Yogurt			
LITE			
plain	8 oz	180	110
strawberry	8 oz	110	200

	Portion	Sodium (mg)	Calories
vanilla	8 oz	130	160
WHOLE MILK			
plain	8 oz	160	150
banana strawberry	8 oz	160	235
blueberry	8 oz	160	250
French vanilla	8 oz	140	210
peach	8 oz	160	230
strawberry	8 oz	160	230
strawberry vanilla	8 oz	160	260
Dannon			
EXTRA SMOOTH YOGURT			
plain	8 oz	160	110
mixed berries, raspberry, or strawberry	4.4 oz	80	130
FRESH FLAVORS YOGURT			
blueberry, raspberry, strawberry, or strawberry banana	8 oz	160	200
coffee, lemon, or vanilla	8 oz	140	200
FRUIT-ON-THE-BOTTOM YOGURT			
all flavors	8 oz	120	240
HEARTY NUTS & RAISINS YOGURT			
plain	8 oz	160	140
mixed berries or orchard fruit	8 oz	120	260
vanilla	8 oz	120	270
Friendship			
buttermilk, low-fat (1½% milk fat)	1 c	125	120
Lite Delite low-fat sour cream	2 T	25	35
sour cream	2 T	15	55
yogurt			
regular (3½% milk fat), plain	1 c	160	170
low-fat (1½% milk fat)			
vanilla & coffee	1 c	170	210
w/fruit	1 c	160	230
Rich's Nondairy Creamers			
Coffee Rich	½ oz	11	22
Poly Rich	½ oz	7	22
Richwhip			
liquid	¼ oz or 1 fl oz whipped	4	20
pressurized	¼ oz	3	20
prewhipped	1 T whipped	1	12

❑ **MOLASSES** *See* SUGARS & SWEETENERS

	Portion	Sodium (mg)	Calories

□ **MUFFINS** *See* BREADS, ROLLS, BISCUITS, & MUFFINS

□ **NOODLES & PASTA, PLAIN**

Noodles

	Portion	Sodium (mg)	Calories
chow funn, dry (Oriental wheat noodles)	1 oz	260	102
chow mein, canned	1 c	450	220
egg, enriched, cooked	1 c	3	200
Japanese style, seasoned *See* Nissin, *under* SOUPS, PREPARED			
saimin, dry (Oriental wheat noodles)	1 oz	261	95

Pasta

	Portion	Sodium (mg)	Calories
macaroni, enriched, cooked (cut lengths, elbows, shells)			
firm stage, hot	1 c	1	190
tender stage			
cold	1 c	1	115
hot	1 c	1	155
prepared & SEASONED PASTA DISHES			
SEE DINNERS, FROZEN; ENTREES & MAIN COURSES, CANNED & BOXED; ENTREES & MAIN COURSES, FROZEN			
spaghetti, enriched, cooked			
firm stage, hot	1 c	1	190
tender stage, hot	1 c	1	155

▪ **BRAND NAME**

Contadina Fresh Cut Pasta
EGG

	Portion	Sodium (mg)	Calories
angel's hair, fettucine, or linguine	4.5 oz	35	370

SPINACH

	Portion	Sodium (mg)	Calories
angel's hair, fettucine, or linguine	4.5 oz	105	370
Health Valley			
elbows			
whole-wheat	2 oz dry	10	197
whole-wheat w/4 vegetables	2 oz dry	10	197
lasagna, whole-wheat	2 oz dry	10	205

	Portion	Sodium (mg)	Calories
spaghetti			
whole-wheat	2 oz dry	10	205
whole-wheat w/amaranth	2 oz dry	10	197
whole-wheat w/spinach	2 oz dry	10	170
spinach lasagna, whole-wheat	2 oz dry	15	200
Mueller's			
egg noodles	2 oz dry	10	220
lasagna	2 oz dry	0	210
spaghetti & macaroni	2 oz dry	0	210
tricolor twists	2 oz dry	20	210

❏ NUTS & NUT-BASED BUTTERS, FLOURS, MEALS, MILKS, PASTES, & POWDERS

See also SEEDS & SEED-BASED BUTTERS, FLOURS, & MEALS

	Portion	Sodium (mg)	Calories
acorns			
dried	1 oz	0	145
raw	1 oz	0	105
almond butter			
plain	1 T	2	101
honey & cinnamon	1 T	2	96
almond meal, partially defatted	1 oz	2	116
almond paste	1 oz	3	127
	1 c firmly packed	21	1,012
almond powder			
full-fat	1 oz	2	168
	1 c not packed	4	385
partially defatted	1 oz	3	112
	1 c not packed	6	255
almonds			
dried			
blanched	1 oz	3	166
	1 c whole kernels	15	850
unblanched	1 oz	3	167
	1 c whole kernels	15	837
dry-roasted, unblanched	1 oz	3	167
	1 c whole kernels	15	810

	Portion	Sodium (mg)	Calories
almonds *(cont.)*			
oil-roasted			
blanched	1 oz	3	174
	1 c whole ker-nels	17	870
unblanched	1 oz	3	176
	1 c whole ker-nels	16	970
toasted, unblanched	1 oz	3	167
Brazil nuts, dried, unblanched	1 oz	0	186
	1 c	2	919
butternuts, dried	1 oz	0	174
cashew butter, plain	1 T	2	94
cashew nuts			
dry-roasted	1 oz	4	163
	1 c wholes & halves	21	787
oil-roasted	1 oz	5	163
	1 c wholes & halves	22	748
chestnuts, Chinese			
raw	1 oz	1	64
boiled, steamed	1 oz	1	44
dried	1 oz	2	103
roasted	1 oz	1	68
chestnuts, European			
raw			
peeled	1 oz	1	56
unpeeled	1 oz	1	60
	1 c	4	308
boiled, steamed	1 oz	8	37
dried			
peeled	1 oz	11	105
unpeeled	1 oz	11	106
roasted	1 oz	1	70
	1 c	3	350
chestnuts, Japanese			
raw	1 oz	4	44
boiled, steamed	1 oz	1	16
dried	1 oz	10	102
	1 c	52	558
coconut cream			
raw	1 T	1	49
	1 c	10	792
canned	1 T	10	36
	1 c	149	568
coconut meat			
raw	1.6 oz	9	159
	1 c shredded or grated	16	283

	Portion	Sodium (mg)	Calories
dried (desiccated)			
creamed	1 oz	11	194
sweetened, flaked, canned	4 oz	23	505
	1 c	15	341
sweetened, flaked, packaged	7 oz	509	944
	1 c	189	351
sweetened, shredded	7 oz	522	997
	1 c	244	466
toasted	1 oz	11	168
unsweetened	1 oz	11	187
coconut milk			
raw	1 T	2	35
	1 c	37	552
canned	1 T	2	30
	1 c	29	445
frozen	1 T	2	30
	1 c	29	486
coconut water	1 T	16	3
	1 c	252	46
filberts or hazelnuts			
dried			
blanched	1 oz	1	191
unblanched	1 oz	1	179
	1 c chopped kernels	3	727
dry-roasted, unblanched	1 oz	1	188
oil-roasted, unblanched	1 oz	1	187
formulated nuts, wheat-based			
unflavored	1 oz	143	177
macadamia-flavored	1 oz	13	176
all other flavors	1 oz	26	184
ginkgo nuts			
raw	1 oz	2	52
canned	1 oz	87	32
	1 c	476	173
dried	1 oz	4	99
hazelnuts *See* filberts, *above*			
hickory nuts, dried	1 oz	0	187
macadamia nuts			
dried	1 oz	1	199
	1 c	6	940
oil-roasted	1 oz	2	204
	1 c wholes or halves	9	962
mixed nuts (cashew nuts, almonds, filberts, & pecans)			
dry-roasted, w/peanuts	1 oz	3	169
	1 c	16	814
oil-roasted			
w/peanuts	1 oz	3	175
	1 c	16	876

	Portion	Sodium (mg)	Calories
peanut butter, w/added fat, sugar, & salt			
chunk style	2 T	156	188
smooth style	2 T	153	188
peanut flour			
low-fat	1 c	0	257
defatted	1 T	50	13
	1 c	108	196
peanuts			
other types			
raw	1 oz	5	159
	1 c	27	828
boiled	½ c	240	102
dried	1 oz	5	161
dry-roasted	1 oz	228	164
	1 c	1,187	855
oil-roasted	1 oz	121	163
	1 c	624	837
Spanish, oil-roasted	1 oz	121	162
	1 c	637	851
Valencia, oil-roasted	1 oz	216	165
	1 c	1,111	848
Virginia, oil-roasted	1 oz	121	161
	1 c	619	826
pecan flour	1 oz	0	93
pecans			
dried	1 oz	0	190
	1 c halves	1	721
dry-roasted	1 oz	0	187
oil-roasted	1 oz	0	195
	1 c	1	754
pignolias *See* pine nuts, *below*			
pili nuts, dried	1 oz	1	204
	1 c	4	863
pine nuts			
pignolia, dried	1 oz	1	146
	1 T	0	51
piñon, dried	1 oz	20	161
	10 kernels	1	6
pistachios			
dried	1 oz	2	164
	1 c	7	739
dry-roasted	1 oz	2	172
	1 c	8	776
sweet chestnuts *See* chestnuts, European, *above*			
walnuts			
black, dried	1 oz	0	172
	1 c chopped	2	759
English or Persian, dried	1 oz	3	182
	1 c pieces	12	770

	Portion	Sodium (mg)	Calories
■ BRAND NAME			
Arrowhead Mills			
peanut butter, creamy or chunky	2 T	2	190
Blue Diamond			
almonds			
raw, whole, unblanched	1 oz	tr	173
blanched, sliced	1 oz	1	176
blanched, whole, raw	1 oz	1	174
dry-roasted, unsalted	1 oz	1	168
oil-roasted, salted	1 oz	95	174
hazelnuts			
raw, whole, Oregon	1 oz	1	166
oil-roasted, salted	1 oz	39	180
pistachios, dry-roasted, salted, natural, California	1 oz	173	162
Erewhon			
almond butter	1 T	18	90
peanut butter			
chunky or creamy, salted	2 T	77	190
chunky or creamy, unsalted	2 T	10	190
Fearn			
Brazil nut burger mix	¼ c dry or ⅛ of 7.6 oz box	230	100
Featherweight			
low-sodium peanut butter			
chunky	1 oz	<3	90
creamy	1 oz	<3	180
Planters			
almonds			
blanched: slivered, whole, or sliced	1 oz	0	170
dry-roasted	1 oz	200	170
honey-roasted	1 oz	180	170
cashews			
dry-roasted			
regular	1 oz	230	230
unsalted	1 oz	0	230
honey-roasted	1 oz	170	170
oil-roasted, fancy or halves			
regular	1 oz	135	170
unsalted	1 oz	0	170
cashews & peanuts, honey-roasted	1 oz	170	170
mixed nuts			
dry-roasted			
regular	1 oz	250	160
unsalted	1 oz	0	170

	Portion	Sodium (mg)	Calories
mixed nuts *(cont.)*			
oil-roasted			
regular	1 oz	130	180
deluxe	1 oz	135	180
unsalted	1 oz	0	180
nut topping	1 oz	0	180
peanuts			
cocktail, oil-roasted			
regular	1 oz	160	170
unsalted	1 oz	0	170
dry-roasted			
regular	1 oz	250	160
unsalted	1 oz	0	170
honey-roasted			
regular	1 oz	180	170
dry-roasted	1 oz	90	160
oil-roasted, salted	1 oz	160	170
redskin, oil-roasted	1 oz	150	170
roasted-in-shell			
salted	1 oz	160	160
unsalted	1 oz	0	160
Spanish			
raw	1 oz	0	150
dry-roasted	1 oz	200	160
oil-roasted	1 oz	150	170
Sweet 'n Crunchy	1 oz	20	140
pecans: chips, halves, or pieces	1 oz	0	190
pistachios			
natural	1 oz	250	170
dry-roasted	1 oz	250	170
red	1 oz	250	170
sesame nut mix			
dry-roasted	1 oz	330	160
oil-roasted	1 oz	220	160
sunflower nuts			
dry-roasted			
regular	1 oz	260	160
unsalted	1 oz	0	170
oil-roasted	1 oz	130	170
Tavern Nuts	1 oz	65	170
walnuts			
black	1 oz	0	180
English: whole, halves, or pieces	1 oz	0	190
Skippy Peanut Butter			
creamy	1 T	75	95
	2 T	150	190
Super Chunk	1 T	65	95
	2 T	130	190

	Portion	Sodium (mg)	Calories
Smucker's			
natural peanut butter	2 T	125	200

❑ **OILS** *See* FATS, OILS, & SHORTENINGS

❑ **OLIVES** *See* PICKLES, OLIVES, RELISHES, & CHUTNEYS

❑ **PASTA** *See* NOODLES & PASTA, PLAIN

❑ **PASTRIES** *See* DESSERTS: CAKES, PASTRIES, & PIES

❑ **PÂTÉS** *See* PROCESSED MEAT & POULTRY PRODUCTS

❑ **PEANUT BUTTER** *See* NUTS & NUT-BASED BUTTERS, FLOURS, MEALS, MILKS, PASTES, & POWDERS

❑ **PICKLES, OLIVES, RELISHES, & CHUTNEYS**
See also peppers; sauerkraut, *under* VEGETABLES, PLAIN & PREPARED

Chutneys

apple	1 T	34	41
tomato	1 T	26	31

Olives, Canned

green	4 medium or 3 extra large	312	15
ripe, Mission, pitted	3 small or 2 large	68	15

	Portion	Sodium (mg)	Calories
Pickles, Cucumber			
bread & butter	4 slices	168	18
dill, whole	1 medium = about 2¼ oz	928	5
fresh-pack	2 slices = about ½ oz	101	10
kosher	1	581	7
sour	1 large	1,353	10
sweet	1 large	572	146
sweet & sour, sliced	1 slice	25	3
sweet gherkin, small, whole	1 = about ½ oz	107	20
Relishes			
cranberry-orange	1 T	tr	27
canned	½ c	44	246
pickle			
chow chow			
sweet	1 oz	148	32
sour	1 oz	375	8
sweet, finely chopped	1 T	107	20
strawberry	1 T	2	53
strawberry-pineapple	1 T	3	54
tomato	1 T	19	53
▪ BRAND NAME			
Claussen			
bread & butter pickle slices	1	61	7
dill pickle spears	1	373	4
kosher pickle halves	1	769	9
kosher pickle slices	1	107	1
kosher tomatoes	1	571	9
kosher whole pickles	1	832	9
no-garlic dills	1	895	17
pickle relish	1 T	90	14
Dromedary			
pimientos, all types, drained	1 oz	5	10
Vlasic			
relishes, hamburger or hot dog	1 oz	255	varies
ONIONS			
lightly spiced cocktail onions	1 oz	370	4
PEPPERS			
hot banana pepper rings	1 oz	470	4
Mexican jalapeño peppers	1 oz	380	8
mild cherry peppers	1 oz	410	8
mild Greek pepperoncini	1 oz	450	4

	Portion	Sodium (mg)	Calories
PICKLES, CUCUMBER			
bread & butter sweet butter chips	1 oz	160	30
Half-the-Salt hamburger dill chips	1 oz	180	2
Hot & Spicy Garden Mix	1 oz	380	4
kosher baby dills	1 oz	210	4
kosher crunchy dills	1 oz	210	4
kosher dill gherkins	1 oz	210	4
refrigerated pickles			
Deli dill halves	1 oz	290	4
dill bread & butter	1 oz	120	25
Zesty crunchy dills	1 oz	250	4
RELISHES			
dill relish	1 oz	420	2
hamburger relish	1 oz	260	40
hot dog relish	1 oz	260	40
sweet relish	1 oz	220	30

❑ PIE FILLINGS *See* DESSERTS: CUSTARDS, GELATINS, PUDDINGS, & PIE FILLINGS

❑ PIES *See* DESSERTS: CAKES, PASTRIES, & PIES

❑ PIZZA

	Portion	Sodium (mg)	Calories
pizza, cheese	⅛ pizza (15″ diam)	699	290

▪ BRAND NAME

	Portion	Sodium (mg)	Calories
Celentano			
9-slice pizza	⅑ pizza = 2.67 oz	166	157
thick crust pizza	⅓ pizza = 4.3 oz	252	238
Celeste Frozen Pizza			
Canadian-style bacon	7¾ oz pizza	1,593	541
	¼ of 19 oz pizza	976	329

	Portion	Sodium (mg)	Calories
cheese	6½ oz pizza	828	497
	¼ of 17¾ oz pizza	673	317
deluxe	8¼ oz pizza	1,308	582
	¼ of 22¼ oz pizza	953	378
pepperoni	6¾ oz pizza	1,417	546
	¼ of 19 oz pizza	1,061	368
sausage	7½ oz pizza	1,374	571
	¼ of 20 oz pizza	988	376
sausage & mushroom	8½ oz pizza	1,347	592
	¼ of 22½ oz pizza	1,033	387
Suprema	9 oz pizza	1,693	678
	¼ of 23 oz pizza	1,043	381
Pepperidge Farm Croissant Pastry Pizza			
cheese	1	730	490
deluxe	1	940	520
hamburger	1	1,040	510
pepperoni	1	810	490
sausage	1	910	540

❑ PORK, FRESH & CURED
See also PROCESSED MEAT & POULTRY PRODUCTS

Pork, Fresh

retail cuts, separable fat, cooked	1 oz	9	200

LEG (HAM)

Lean & Fat

whole, roasted	3 oz	51	250
	1 c	83	411
rump half, roasted	3 oz	52	233
	1 c	85	384
shank half, roasted	3 oz	50	258
	1 c	82	425

Lean Only

whole, roasted	3 oz	55	187
	1 c	90	309
rump half, roasted	3 oz	55	187
	1 c	90	309
shank half, roasted	3 oz	54	183
	1 c	90	301

	Portion	Sodium (mg)	Calories
LOIN, WHOLE			
Lean & Fat			
braised	3 oz	56	312
	1 chop (3 chops/lb as purchased)	46	261
broiled	3 oz	56	294
	1 chop (3 chops/lb as purchased)	54	284
roasted	3 oz	53	271
	1 chop (3 chops/lb as purchased)	52	262
Lean Only			
braised	3 oz	63	232
	1 chop (3 chops/lb as purchased)	41	150
broiled	3 oz	64	218
	1 chop (3 chops/lb as purchased)	49	169
roasted	3 oz	59	204
	1 chop (3 chops/lb as purchased)	48	166
LOIN, BLADE			
Lean & Fat			
braised	3 oz	59	348
	1 chop (3 chops/lb as purchased)	46	275
broiled	3 oz	57	334
	1 chop (3 chops/lb as purchased)	52	303
pan-fried	3 oz	52	352
	1 chop (3 chops/lb as purchased)	55	368
roasted	3 oz	52	310
	1 chop (3 chops/lb as purchased)	54	321

	Portion	Sodium (mg)	Calories
Lean Only			
braised	3 oz	69	266
	1 chop (3 chops/lb as purchased)	41	156
broiled	3 oz	65	255
	1 chop (3 chops/lb as purchased)	45	177
pan-fried	3 oz	63	240
	1 chop (3 chops/lb as purchased)	46	175
roasted	3 oz	58	238
	1 chop (3 chops/lb as purchased)	48	198
LOIN, CENTER			
Lean & Fat			
braised	3 oz	43	301
	1 chop (3 chops/lb as purchased)	38	266
broiled	3 oz	59	269
	1 chop (3 chops/lb as purchased)	61	275
pan-fried	3 oz	61	318
	1 chop (3 chops/lb as purchased)	64	333
roasted	3 oz	54	259
	1 chop (3 chops/lb as purchased)	56	268
Lean Only			
braised	3 oz	46	231
	1 chop (3 chops/lb as purchased)	33	166
broiled	3 oz	66	196
	1 chop (3 chops/lb as purchased)	56	166

	Portion	Sodium (mg)	Calories
pan-fried	3 oz	72	226
	1 chop (3 chops/lb as purchased)	57	178
roasted	3 oz	59	204
	1 chop (3 chops/lb as purchased)	52	180

LOIN, CENTER RIB
Lean & Fat

braised	3 oz	41	312
	1 chop (3 chops/lb as purchased)	32	246
broiled	3 oz	52	291
	1 chop (3 chops/lb as purchased)	47	264
pan-fried	3 oz	38	331
	1 chop (3 chops/lb as purchased)	40	343
roasted	3 oz	37	271
	1 chop (3 chops/lb as purchased)	35	252

Lean Only

braised	3 oz	44	236
	1 chop (3 chops/lb as purchased)	28	147
broiled	3 oz	57	219
	1 chop (3 chops/lb as purchased)	42	162
pan-fried	3 oz	43	219
	1 chop (3 chops/lb as purchased)	31	160
roasted	3 oz	39	208
	1 chop (3 chops/lb as purchased)	30	162

	Portion	Sodium (mg)	Calories
LOIN, SIRLOIN			
Lean & Fat			
braised	3 oz	45	299
	1 chop (3 chops/lb as purchased)	38	250
broiled	3 oz	46	281
	1 chop (3 chops/lb as purchased)	46	278
roasted	3 oz	50	247
	1 chop (3 chops/lb as purchased)	49	244
Lean Only			
braised	3 oz	50	221
	1 chop (3 chops/lb as purchased)	34	149
broiled	3 oz	51	207
	1 chop (3 chops/lb as purchased)	41	165
roasted	3 oz	53	201
	1 chop (3 chops/lb as purchased)	46	175
LOIN, TENDERLOIN			
lean, roasted	3 oz	57	141
LOIN, TOP			
Lean & Fat			
braised	3 oz	40	324
	1 chop (3 chops/lb as purchased)	33	267
broiled	3 oz	51	306
	1 chop (3 chops/lb as purchased)	49	295
pan-fried	3 oz	38	333
	1 chop (3 chops/lb as purchased)	39	337

	Portion	Sodium (mg)	Calories
roasted	3 oz	37	280
	1 chop (3 chops/lb as purchased)	36	274
Lean Only			
braised	3 oz	44	236
	1 chop (3 chops/lb as purchased)	28	147
broiled	3 oz	57	219
	1 chop (3 chops/lb as purchased)	43	165
pan-fried	3 oz	43	219
	1 chop (3 chops/lb as purchased)	31	157
roasted	3 oz	39	208
	1 chop (3 chops/lb as purchased)	31	167
SHOULDER, WHOLE			
lean & fat, roasted	3 oz	58	277
	1 c	96	456
lean only, roasted	3 oz	65	207
	1 c	107	341
SHOULDER, ARM PICNIC			
Lean & Fat			
braised	3 oz	74	293
	1 c	123	483
roasted	3 oz	59	281
	1 c	97	463
Lean Only			
braised	3 oz	87	211
	1 c	143	347
roasted	3 oz	68	194
	1 c	112	319
SHOULDER, BLADE, BOSTON			
Lean & Fat			
braised	3 oz	57	316
	1 steak	107	594
broiled	3 oz	63	297
	1 steak	138	647
roasted	3 oz	57	273
	1 steak	125	594

	Portion	Sodium (mg)	Calories
Lean Only			
braised	3 oz	64	250
	1 steak	98	382
broiled	3 oz	71	233
	1 steak	126	413
roasted	3 oz	62	218
	1 steak	116	404
SPARERIBS			
lean & fat, braised	3 oz	79	338
	6¼ oz (yield from 1 lb as purchased)	165	703
VARIETY MEATS			
brains, braised	3 oz	77	117
chitterlings, simmered	3 oz	33	258
ears, simmered	1	183	183
heart, braised	1	46	191
kidneys, braised	1 c	111	211
liver, braised	3 oz	42	141
lungs, braised	3 oz	68	84
tongue, braised	3 oz	93	230

Pork, Cured

	Portion	Sodium (mg)	Calories
bacon, pan-fried or roasted	3 medium slices (20 slices/lb)	303	109
breakfast strips, cooked	3 slices (15 slices/12 oz)	714	156
	6 oz	3,568	780
Canadian-style bacon, unheated, fully cooked as purchased	2 oz	799	89
ham, whole			
lean & fat			
unheated, fully cooked as	1 oz	364	70
purchased	1 c	1,797	345
roasted	3 oz	1,009	207
	1 c	1,661	341
lean only			
unheated, fully cooked as	1 oz	430	42
purchased	1 c	2,122	206
roasted	3 oz	1,128	133
	1 c	1,858	219

	Portion	Sodium (mg)	Calories
ham, boneless			
regular (about 11% fat)			
unheated	1 oz	373	52
	1 c	1,844	255
roasted	3 oz	1,275	151
	1 c	2,100	249
extra lean (about 5% fat)			
unheated	1 oz	405	37
	1 c	2,000	183
roasted	3 oz	1,023	123
	1 c	1,684	203
ham, canned			
regular (about 13% fat)			
unheated	1 oz	352	54
	1 c	1,736	266
roasted	3 oz	800	192
	1 c	1,317	317
extra lean (about 4% fat)			
unheated	1 oz	356	34
	1 c	1,757	168
roasted	3 oz	965	116
	1 c	1,589	191
ham, center slice			
lean & fat, unheated, fully	4 oz	1,566	229
cooked as purchased	1 oz	393	57
ham patties			
grilled	2 oz	632	203
unheated, fully cooked as	2.3 oz	709	206
purchased			
ham steak, boneless, extra	2 oz	720	69
lean, unheated, fully			
cooked as purchased			
salt pork, raw	1 oz	404	212
separable fat (from ham & arm picnic)			
unheated, fully cooked as	1 oz	143	164
purchased			
roasted	1 oz	177	167
shoulder			
arm picnic, roasted			
lean & fat	3 oz	912	238
	1 c	1,501	392
lean only	3 oz	1,046	145
	1 c	1,723	238
blade roll, lean & fat			
unheated, fully cooked as	1 oz	354	76
purchased			
roasted	3 oz	827	244

	Portion	Sodium (mg)	Calories
▪ BRAND NAME			
Armour & Armour Star			
BACON			
1877 Canadian bacon	2 oz	850	80
lower-salt bacon			
raw	1 slice = 0.3 oz	127	38
cooked	1 slice = 0.2 oz	100	30
sliced bacon	1 slice = 0.9 oz	180	130
thick-sliced bacon	1 slice = 1.3 oz	265	190
HAM			
boneless, cooked, lower salt, 93% fat-free	1 oz	242	41
canned	1 oz	354	34
chopped	3 oz	1,100	260
Golden Star, canned	3 oz	970	90
Speedy Cut, boneless, cooked	1 oz	330	44
Oscar Mayer			
BACON & BREAKFAST STRIPS			
bacon	1 cooked slice	118	35
Bacon Bits	¼ oz	181	21
breakfast strips, pork	1 strip, raw	215	54
Canadian-style bacon	1 oz	389	35
thick-sliced bacon	1 cooked slice	208	64
HAM			
boneless Jubilee ham	1 oz	369	46
chopped ham	1 oz	327	55
cracked black pepper ham	¾ oz	296	24
honey ham	¾ oz	276	26
Jubilee canned ham	1 oz	285	31
Jubilee ham slice	1 oz	352	29
Jubilee ham steaks	2 oz	717	59
smoked cooked ham	2 oz	268	23

	Portion	Sodium (mg)	Calories

❏ POULTRY, FRESH & PROCESSED
See also PROCESSED MEAT & POULTRY PRODUCTS

NOTE: Values are based on the following weights as purchased with giblets & neck:

chicken	
broilers or fryers	3.33 lbs
roasting	4.56 lbs
stewing	2.93 lbs
capons	6.5 lbs

duck	
domesticated	4.42 lbs
wild	2.26 lbs
goose	8.25 lbs
guinea	1.92 lbs
pheasant	2.15 lbs
quail	0.27 lb
squab	0.67 lb

turkey	
all classes	15.47 lbs
fryer-roasters	7.05 lbs
young hens	12.54 lbs
young toms	23.06 lbs

Chicken, Fresh

CHICKEN, BROILERS OR FRYERS

	Portion	Sodium (mg)	Calories
flesh, skin, giblets, & neck			
fried			
batter-dipped	1 chicken	2,921	2,987
flour-coated	1 chicken	606	1,928
roasted	1 chicken	536	1,598
stewed	1 chicken	494	1,625
flesh & skin			
fried			
batter-dipped	½ chicken	1,360	1,347
flour-coated	½ chicken	264	844
roasted	½ chicken	244	715
stewed	½ chicken	224	730
flesh only			
fried	1 c	127	307
roasted	1 c	120	266
stewed	1 c	98	248

	Portion	Sodium (mg)	Calories
skin only			
fried			
batter-dipped	½ chicken	1,105	748
flour-coated	½ chicken	30	281
roasted	½ chicken	36	254
stewed	½ chicken	40	261
giblets			
fried, flour-coated	1 c	164	402
simmered	1 c	85	228
gizzard, simmered	1 c	97	222
heart, simmered	1 c	69	268
liver, simmered	1 c	71	219
light meat w/skin			
fried			
batter-dipped	½ chicken	539	520
flour-coated	½ chicken	100	320
roasted	½ chicken	99	293
stewed	½ chicken	95	302
dark meat w/skin			
fried			
batter-dipped	½ chicken	821	828
flour-coated	½ chicken	164	523
roasted	½ chicken	145	423
stewed	½ chicken	129	428
light meat w/out skin			
fried	1 c	114	268
roasted	1 c	108	242
stewed	1 c	91	223
dark meat w/out skin			
fried	1 c	136	334
roasted	1 c	130	286
stewed	1 c	104	269
back, meat & skin			
fried			
batter-dipped	½ back	380	397
flour-coated	½ back	65	238
roasted	½ back	46	159
stewed	½ back	39	158
back, meat only			
fried	½ back	58	167
roasted	½ back	38	96
stewed	½ back	28	88
breast, meat & skin			
fried			
batter-dipped	½ breast	385	364
flour-coated	½ breast	75	218
roasted	½ breast	69	193
stewed	½ breast	68	202
breast, meat only			
fried	½ breast	68	161

	Portion	Sodium (mg)	Calories
roasted	½ breast	63	142
stewed	½ breast	59	144
drumstick, meat & skin			
fried			
batter-dipped	1	194	193
flour-coated	1	44	120
roasted	1	47	112
stewed	1	43	116
drumstick, meat only			
fried	1	40	82
roasted	1	42	76
stewed	1	37	78
leg (drumstick & thigh), meat & skin			
fried			
batter-dipped	1	442	431
flour-coated	1	99	285
roasted	1	99	265
stewed	1	92	275
leg (drumstick & thigh), meat only			
fried	1	90	195
roasted	1	87	182
stewed	1	78	187
neck, meat & skin			
fried			
batter-dipped	1	143	172
flour-coated	1	29	119
simmered	1	20	94
neck, meat only			
fried	1	22	50
simmered	1	12	32
thigh, meat & skin			
fried			
batter-dipped	1	248	238
flour-coated	1	55	162
roasted	1	52	153
stewed	1	49	158
thigh, meat only			
fried	1	49	113
roasted	1	46	109
stewed	1	41	107
wing, meat & skin			
fried			
batter-dipped	1	157	159
flour-coated	1	25	103
roasted	1	28	99
stewed	1	27	100
wing, meat only			
fried	1	18	42

	Portion	Sodium (mg)	Calories
wing, meat only *(cont.)*			
roasted	1	19	43
stewed	1	18	43
CHICKEN, ROASTING			
flesh & skin, roasted	½ chicken	349	1,071
flesh only, roasted	1 c	105	233
giblets, simmered	1 c	86	239
light meat w/out skin, roasted	1 c	71	214
dark meat w/out skin, roasted	1 c	133	250
CHICKEN, STEWING			
flesh, skin, giblets, & neck, stewed	1 chicken	419	1,636
flesh & skin, stewed	½ chicken	190	744
flesh only, stewed	1 c	109	332
giblets, simmered	1 c	81	281
light meat w/out skin, stewed	1 c	81	298
dark meat w/out skin, stewed	1 c	133	361
CHICKEN, CAPONS			
flesh, skin, giblets, & neck, roasted	1 chicken	704	3,211
flesh & skin, roasted	½ chicken	313	1,457
giblets, simmered	1 c	80	238

Duck, Fresh

DOMESTICATED			
flesh & skin, roasted	½ duck	227	1,287
flesh only, roasted	½ duck	143	445
WILD			
flesh & skin, raw	1 lb of ready-to-cook bird	135	505
breast, meat only, raw	½ breast	47	102

Goose, Fresh, Domesticated

flesh & skin, roasted	½ goose	543	2,362
flesh only, roasted	½ goose	447	1,406
liver, raw	1	132	125

Pheasant, Fresh

flesh & skin, raw	1 lb of ready-to-cook bird	150	670
flesh only, raw	1 lb of ready-to-cook bird	121	435
breast, meat only, raw	½ breast	60	243
leg, meat only, raw	1	48	143

	Portion	Sodium (mg)	Calories

Quail, Fresh

breast, meat only, raw	1	31	69
flesh & skin, raw	1 quail	58	210
flesh only, raw	1 quail	47	123

Turkey, Fresh

TURKEY, ALL CLASSES

flesh, skin, giblets, & neck, roasted	1 lb of ready-to-cook bird	175	533
	1 turkey	2,715	8,245
flesh & skin, roasted	1 lb of ready-to-cook bird	164	498
	½ turkey	1,269	3,857
flesh only, roasted	1 c	99	238
skin only, roasted	½ turkey	132	1,096
giblets, simmered	1 c	85	243
gizzard, simmered	1 c	79	236
heart, simmered	1 c	79	257
liver, simmered	1 c	89	237
light meat w/skin, roasted	½ turkey	658	2,069
dark meat w/skin, roasted	½ turkey	612	1,789
light meat w/out skin, roasted	1 c	89	219
dark meat w/out skin, roasted	1 c	110	262
back, meat & skin, roasted	½ back	191	637
breast, meat & skin, roasted	½ breast	541	1,637
leg, meat & skin, roasted	1	420	1,133
neck, meat only, simmered	1	84	274
wing, meat & skin, roasted	1	114	426

TURKEY, FRYER ROASTERS

flesh, skin, giblets, & neck, roasted	1 lb of ready-to-cook bird	163	429
	1 turkey	1,150	3,029
flesh & skin, roasted	1 lb of ready-to-cook bird	151	395
	½ turkey	532	1,392
flesh only, roasted	1 lb of ready-to-cook bird	130	292
	1 c	94	210
skin only, roasted	1 lb of ready-to-cook bird	21	102
	½ turkey	73	362
light meat w/skin, roasted	½ turkey	247	711
dark meat w/skin, roasted	½ turkey	285	680
light meat w/out skin, roasted	1 c	79	195
dark meat w/out skin, roasted back	1 c	110	227
meat & skin, roasted	½ back	90	265
meat only, roasted	½ back	70	164

	Portion	Sodium (mg)	Calories
breast			
meat & skin, roasted	½ breast	182	526
meat only, roasted	½ breast	159	413
leg			
meat & skin, roasted	1	195	418
meat only, roasted	1	182	355
wing			
meat & skin, roasted	1	65	186
meat only, roasted	1	47	98

TURKEY, YOUNG HENS

	Portion	Sodium (mg)	Calories
flesh, skin, giblets, & neck, roasted	1 lb of ready-to-cook bird	166	565
	1 turkey	2,080	7,094
flesh & skin, roasted	½ turkey	977	3,323
flesh only, roasted	1 c	93	244
skin only, roasted	½ turkey	87	945
light meat w/skin, roasted	½ turkey	501	1,778
dark meat w/skin, roasted	½ turkey	476	1,544
light meat w/out skin, roasted	1 c	84	226
dark meat w/out skin, roasted	1 c	105	268
back, meat & skin, roasted	½ back	149	551
breast, meat & skin, roasted	½ breast	401	1,330
leg, meat & skin, roasted	1	326	955
wing, meat & skin, roasted	1	98	414

TURKEY, YOUNG TOMS

	Portion	Sodium (mg)	Calories
flesh, skin, giblets, & neck, roasted	1 lb of ready-to-cook bird	185	514
	1 turkey	4,279	11,873
flesh & skin, roasted	1 lb of ready-to-cook bird	173	482
	½ turkey	1,993	5,545
flesh only, roasted	1 c	104	235
skin only, roasted	½ turkey	224	1,578
light meat w/skin, roasted	½ turkey	1,051	2,992
dark meat w/skin, roasted	½ turkey	942	2,553
light meat w/out skin, roasted	1 c	95	215
dark meat w/out skin, roasted	1 c	115	260
back, meat & skin			
raw	½ back	392	940
roasted	½ back	294	903
breast, meat & skin, roasted	½ breast	892	2,510
leg, meat & skin, roasted	1	648	1,660
wing, meat & skin, roasted	1	157	524

	Portion	Sodium (mg)	Calories
Poultry, Processed			
MECHANICALLY DEBONED POULTRY			
from broiler backs & necks			
w/skin, raw	½ lb	90	616
w/out skin, raw	½ lb	115	450
TURKEY			
gravy & turkey, frozen	5 oz	786	95
patties, breaded, battered, fried	2¼ oz	512	181
	3⅓ oz	752	266
prebasted turkey			
breast, meat & skin, roasted	½ breast	3,434	1,087
thigh, meat & skin, roasted	1	1,371	494
roasts, boneless, frozen, sea-	0.43 lb	1,334	304
soned, light & dark meat, roasted	1.72 lb	5,320	1,213
sticks, breaded, battered, fried	1 stick = 2¼ oz	536	178

▪ BRAND NAME

Armour & Armour Star

	Portion	Sodium (mg)	Calories
broth-basted turkey, w/ or w/out sugar	4 oz	185	180
butter-basted turkey	4 oz	155	190
turkey roast w/gravy			
white & dark meat	3.69 oz	655	150
white meat only	3.69 oz	655	140
Land O'Lakes			
TURKEY PARTS			
breast	3 oz	55	100
drumsticks	3 oz	85	120
hindquarters roast	3 oz	80	140
thighs	3 oz	75	150
wings	3 oz	65	120
WHOLE TURKEY			
butter-basted young turkey	3 oz	135	140
self-basting (broth) young turkey	3 oz	145	120
young turkey	3 oz	55	130
Tyson			
FULLY COOKED CHICKEN			
Batter Gold	about 3½ oz	312	285
buttermilk	about 3½ oz	500	285
Delecta Delicious	about 3½ oz	496	305

	Portion	Sodium (mg)	Calories
Heat N Serve (oven ready)	about 3½ oz	588	270
Honey Stung	about 3½ oz	622	260
lightly breaded	about 3½ oz	724	255
POULTRY PRODUCTS			
breast strips	about 3½ oz	295	270
chicken pattie	about 3½ oz	364	275
Heat N Serve	about 3½ oz	331	280
Sandwich Mate	about 3½ oz	1,001	315
School Lunch pattie	about 3½ oz	690	290
READY-TO-COOK POULTRY			
boneless breast	about 3½ oz	59	205
Cornish & split Cornish	about 3½ oz	65	240
IQF chicken & split broilers	about 3½ oz	70	245
prebreaded marinated chicken	about 3½ oz	520	285

❏ **POULTRY SPREADS** *See* PROCESSED MEAT & POULTRY PRODUCTS

❏ **PRESERVES** *See* FRUIT SPREADS

❏ **PROCESSED MEAT & POULTRY PRODUCTS: SAUSAGES, FRANKFURTERS, COLD CUTS, PÂTÉS, & SPREADS**
See also BEEF, FRESH & CURED; PORK, FRESH & CURED; POULTRY, FRESH & PROCESSED

	Portion	Sodium (mg)	Calories
bacon & Canadian-style bacon *See* PORK, FRESH & CURED			
barbecue loaf, pork, beef	1 oz	378	49
beef sausage, smoked	1 oz	321	89
	1½ oz	486	134
beerwurst, beer salami			
beef	0.2 oz	56	19
	0.8 oz	214	75
pork	0.2 oz	74	14
	0.8 oz	285	55
berliner, pork, beef	1 oz	368	65
bologna			
beef	0.8 oz	230	72
	1 oz	284	89
beef & pork	0.8 oz	234	73
	1 oz	289	89

	Portion	Sodium (mg)	Calories
pork	0.8 oz	272	57
	1 oz	336	70
turkey	1 oz	249	57
bratwurst, cooked, pork	1 oz	158	85
	3 oz	473	256
braunschweiger (a liver sausage), pork	0.6 oz	206	65
	1 oz	324	102
breakfast strips *See* BEEF, FRESH & CURED; PORK, FRESH & CURED			
brotwurst, pork, beef	1 oz	315	92
	2½ oz	778	226
cheesefurter, pork, beef	1½ oz	465	141
chicken roll, light meat	2 oz	331	90
	6 oz	992	271
chicken, canned, boned, w/ broth	5 oz	714	234
corned beef, braised *See* BEEF, FRESH & CURED			
corned beef, canned	1 oz	285	71
corned beef loaf, jellied	1 oz	294	46
dried beef	1 oz	984	47
Dutch brand loaf, pork, beef	1 oz	354	68
frankfurter			
beef	2 oz	584	184
	1.6 oz	461	145
beef & pork	2 oz	639	183
	1.6 oz	504	144
chicken	1.6 oz	617	116
	1 oz	388	73
turkey	1.6 oz	642	102
	1 oz	404	64
ham, boneless or canned *See* PORK, FRESH & CURED			
ham, chopped	1 oz	389	65
ham, chopped, canned	1 oz	387	68
ham, minced	1 oz	353	75
ham & cheese loaf or roll	1 oz	381	73
ham & cheese spread	1 T	179	37
	1 oz	339	69
ham salad spread	1 T	137	32
	1 oz	259	61
head cheese, pork	1 oz	356	60
honey loaf, pork, beef	1 oz	374	36
honey roll sausage, beef	1 oz	375	52
hot dog *See* frankfurter, *above*			
Italian sausage, pork			
raw	3.2 oz	665	315
	4 oz	826	391
cooked	2.3 oz	618	216
	2.9 oz	765	268
kielbasa, pork, beef	1 oz	305	88
knockwurst, pork, beef	2.4 oz	687	209
	1 oz	286	87

	Portion	Sodium (mg)	Calories
Lebanon bologna, beef	0.8 oz	291	52
	1 oz	359	64
liver cheese, pork	1.3 oz	465	115
	1 oz	347	86
luncheon meat			
beef, jellied	1 oz	375	31
beef, loaved	1 oz	377	87
beef, thin-sliced	1 oz	470	35
pork, beef	1 oz	367	100
pork, canned	1 oz	365	95
luncheon sausage, pork & beef	0.8 oz	272	60
	1 oz	335	74
mortadella, beef, pork	about ½ oz	187	47
	1 oz	353	88
olive loaf, pork	1 oz	421	67
pastrami			
beef	1 oz	348	99
turkey	2 oz	593	80
	8 oz	2,372	320
pâté			
liver (not specified), canned	1 T	91	41
	1 oz	198	90
peppered loaf, pork, beef	1 oz	432	42
pepperoni, pork, beef	8.8 oz	5,120	1,248
	0.2 oz	112	27
pickle & pimento loaf, pork	1 oz	394	74
picnic loaf, pork, beef	1 oz	330	66
Polish sausage, pork	8 oz	1,989	739
	1 oz	248	92
pork & beef sausage, fresh, cooked	about 1 oz	217	107
	about ½ oz	105	52
pork sausage, country style, fresh, cooked	about 1 oz	349	100
	about ½ oz	168	48
salami			
cooked			
beef	0.8 oz	266	58
	1 oz	328	72
beef & pork	0.8 oz	245	57
	1 oz	302	71
turkey	2 oz	569	111
	8 oz	2,278	446
dry or hard			
pork	0.35 oz	226	41
	4 oz	2,554	460
pork, beef	0.35 oz	186	42
	4 oz	2,101	472
sandwich spread			
pork, beef	1 T	152	35
	1 oz	287	67

	Portion	Sodium (mg)	Calories
poultry salad	1 T	49	26
	1 oz	107	57
smoked chopped beef	1 oz	357	38
smoked link sausage			
pork, grilled	2.4 oz	1,020	265
	about ½ oz	240	62
pork & beef	2.4 oz	642	229
	about ½ oz	151	54
flour & nonfat dry milk	2.4 oz	741	182
added	about ½ oz	174	43
nonfat dry milk added	2.4 oz	798	213
	about ½ oz	188	50
Thuringer, cervelat, summer	0.8 oz	334	80
sausage: beef, pork	1 oz	412	98
turkey			
canned, boned, w/broth	5 oz	663	231
diced, light & dark, seasoned	1 oz	241	39
	½ lb	1,928	313
turkey breast meat	0.7 oz	301	23
turkey ham (cured turkey thigh	2 oz	565	73
meat)	8 oz	2,260	291
turkey loaf, breast meat	1½ oz	608	47
	6 oz	2,433	187
turkey pastrami See pastrami: turkey, above			
turkey roll, light & dark meat	1 oz	166	42
turkey roll, light meat	1 oz	139	42
Vienna sausage, canned, beef	0.6 oz	152	45
& pork			

▪ BRAND NAME

Armour & Armour Star
FRANKFURTERS

beef	1.6 oz	455	150
Giant All Meat	1.6 oz	455	150
Giant Beef	1 link	565	180
Giant Great 8 Beef	2 oz	565	180
Giant Great 8 Meat	2 oz	565	180
turkey	2 oz	580	110

LUNCHEON MEATS

barbecue loaf	1 oz	380	50
beef bologna, lower salt	1 oz	190	90
bologna or beef bologna, regular	1 oz	310	100
bologna, lower salt	1 oz	200	90

	Portion	Sodium (mg)	Calories
liverwurst	1 oz	325	90
Old Fashioned Loaf	1 oz	320	80
pepperoni			
Italian	1 oz	500	130
sliced	1 oz	532	130
salami			
cotto	1 oz	308	81
Genoa, sliced	1 oz	475	110
Italian, hard	1 oz	520	120
lower-salt cotto	1 oz	184	77
sliced	1 oz	496	120
spiced luncheon meat			
regular	1 oz	308	81
w/chicken	3 oz	1,040	280
summer sausage, cheese	1 oz	380	100
turkey bologna	1 oz	310	60
turkey ham	1 oz	320	35
turkey pastrami	1 oz	330	40
turkey roll, Magic Slice, cooked			
white	3 oz	685	120
white & dark	3 oz	695	120
MEAT PRODUCTS, CANNED			
corned beef hash	1½ oz	1,430	390
deviled ham	1½ oz	380	110
Deviled Treet	1½ oz	400	120
potted meat	1½ oz	450	80
roast beef hash	7½ oz	1,310	350
sloppy joes, beef	about 7½ oz	1,590	390
smoked Vienna sausage	2 oz	400	180
Vienna sausage in beef stock	2 oz	420	180
SAUSAGES			
Country sausage, uncooked, lower salt	1 oz	115	98
sausage links, uncooked, lower salt	1 oz	115	98
sausage patties, uncooked, lower salt	1½ oz	173	147
Carl Buddig Luncheon Meats			
beef	1 oz	430	40
chicken	1 oz	340	60
corned beef	1 oz	380	40
ham	1 oz	400	50
pastrami	1 oz	320	40
turkey	1 oz	400	50
turkey ham	1 oz	430	40
turkey pastrami	1 oz	440	40

	Portion	Sodium (mg)	Calories
Health Valley			
bologna			
beef, sliced	1 slice	321	85
chicken	1 slice	329	85
frankfurters			
beef	1 weiner	109	96
chicken	1 weiner	90	96
turkey	1 weiner	112	96
knockwurst	1 weiner	319	96
Louis Rich			
barbecued breast of turkey	1 oz	305	36
ground turkey	1 cooked oz	29	61
hickory smoked breast of turkey	1 oz	363	31
oven-roasted breast of turkey	1 oz	284	30
oven-roasted chicken breast	1 oz	107	39
smoked turkey breast, sliced	¾ oz	196	21
turkey breast	1 cooked oz	20	50
turkey franks	1 link = 1.58 oz	488	103
turkey ham	1 oz	283	34
turkey pastrami	1 oz	279	33
turkey salami	1 oz	247	52
turkey smoked sausage	1 oz	234	55
Oscar Mayer			
FRANKFURTERS			
beef	1 link	460	144
cheese	1 link	486	145
little wieners	1 link	92	28
wieners	1 link	460	144
LUNCHEON MEATS			
Bar-B-Q loaf	1 oz	346	48
beef bologna	1 oz	311	90
beef cotto salami	0.8 oz	298	46
beef salami for beer	0.8 oz	279	66
beef summer sausage	0.8 oz	327	72
bologna	1 oz	303	90
braunschweiger liver sausage	1 oz	327	96
corned beef	0.6 oz	208	16
cotto salami	0.8 oz	291	54
Genoa salami	0.3 oz	164	34
German brand braunschweiger	1 oz	345	94
ham *See* PORK, FRESH & CURED			
ham & cheese loaf	1 oz	360	76
hard salami	0.3 oz	169	34
head cheese	1 oz	347	55
honey loaf	1 oz	365	35
liver cheese	1.3 oz	432	116

	Portion	Sodium (mg)	Calories
luncheon meat	1 oz	333	98
Luxury Loaf	1 oz	300	38
New England brand sausage	0.8 oz	293	31
Old Fashioned Loaf	1 oz	334	64
olive loaf	1 oz	402	62
pastrami	0.6 oz	219	16
peppered loaf	1 oz	361	43
pickle & pimiento loaf	1 oz	394	63
picnic loaf	1 oz	334	62
summer sausage	0.8 oz	332	73
SAUSAGES			
Beef Smokies	1 link	430	123
Little Friers, pork	1 link	219	82
Little Smokies	1 link	91	28
Smokie Links	1 link	435	124
SLICED CHICKEN & TURKEY			
smoked chicken breast	1 oz	405	26
smoked turkey breast	0.7 oz	268	23
SPREADS			
braunschweiger liver sausage	1 oz	321	96
ham & cheese	1 oz	323	67
ham salad	1 oz	268	59
sandwich	1 oz	268	67
Swanson			
chunk premium white chicken, canned	2½ oz	240	100
chunk white & dark chicken, canned	2½ oz	240	100
chunk-style Mixin' Chicken, canned	2½ oz	230	130
chunky chicken spread	1 oz	140	60
Tyson			
all-white cooked chicken fryer meat	about 3½ oz	64	166
breast of chicken roll, whole & diced	about 3 oz	481	150
chicken bologna	about 3½ oz	1,000	230
chicken corn dogs	about 3½ oz	1,062	280
chicken franks	about 3½ oz	1,180	285
Liberty Roll, whole & diced	about 3½ oz	697	185
natural proportioned cooked chicken meat	about 3½ oz	75	170

□ **PUDDING DESSERTS, FROZEN**
See DESSERTS, FROZEN

	Portion	Sodium (mg)	Calories

❏ PUDDINGS & PIE FILLINGS
See DESSERTS: CUSTARDS, GELATINS, PUDDINGS, & PIE FILLINGS

❏ RELISHES *See* PICKLES, OLIVES, RELISHES, & CHUTNEYS

❏ RICE & GRAINS, PLAIN & PREPARED
See also VEGETABLES, PLAIN & PREPARED

	Portion	Sodium (mg)	Calories
barley, pearled, light, uncooked	1 c	6	700
bulgur, uncooked	1 c	7	600
hominy grits *See* corn grits, *under* BREAKFAST CEREALS, COLD & HOT			
popcorn *See* SNACKS			
rice			
brown, cooked, hot	1 c	0	230
white, enriched			
raw	1 c	9	670
cooked, hot	1 c	0	225
instant, ready-to-serve, hot	1 c	0	180
parboiled, raw	1 c	17	685
parboiled, cooked, hot	1 c	0	185

▪ BRAND NAME

Arrowhead Mills
PLAIN RICE & GRAINS

	Portion	Sodium (mg)	Calories
barley, pearled, or barley flakes	2 oz	2	200
buckwheat groats, brown or white	2 oz	2	190
bulgur wheat	2 oz	0	200
corn, blue	2 oz	2	210
millet	2 oz	1	90
oat flakes	2 oz	1	220
oat groats	2 oz	1	220
quinoa	2 oz	5	200
rice, brown: long, long basmati, medium, or short	2 oz	5	200
triticale or triticale flakes	2 oz	1	190
wheat, hard, red, winter, or soft pastry	2 oz	2	190
wheat flakes	2 oz	2	210

	Portion	Sodium (mg)	Calories
PREPARED RICE & GRAINS			
quick brown rice			
regular	2 oz	2	200
Spanish style	¼ of 5.65 oz pkg	255	150
vegetable herb	¼ of 5.6 oz pkg	150	150
wild rice & herbs	¼ of 5.35 oz pkg	220	140
Birds Eye International Rice Recipes			
French style	3.3 oz	610	110
Italian style	3.3 oz	350	120
Spanish style	3.3 oz	540	110
Carolina Rice			
extra-long grain, enriched	about ½ c cooked	<10	100
Chun King			
rice mix	¼ oz	310	20
Fearn			
Naturfresh corn germ	¼ c or 1 oz	1	130
Naturfresh raw wheat germ	¼ c or 1 oz	1	100
Featherweight			
Spanish rice	7½ oz	32	140
Health Valley			
amaranth pilaf			
regular	4 oz	427	210
no salt	4 oz	15	100
Mahatma			
long grain rice, enriched	about ½ c cooked	<10	100
natural long grain rice, brown	about ½ c cooked	<10	110
Minute Rice			
drumstick mix, w/salted butter	½ c	690	150
fried rice mix, w/oil	½ c	550	160
long grain & wild rice mix, w/ salted	½ c	570	150
rib roast mix, w/salted butter	½ c	720	150
rice, w/out salt or butter	⅔ c	0	120
Pillsbury Frozen Rice Originals			
Italian blend white rice & spinach in cheese sauce	½ c	400	170
long grain white & wild rice	½ c	550	120
rice & broccoli in flavored cheese	½ c	510	120

	Portion	Sodium (mg)	Calories
Rice Jubilee	½ c	340	150
Rice Medley	½ c	260	120
rice pilaf	½ c	520	120
rice w/herb butter sauce	½ c	390	150
Quaker Oats			
Scotch brand medium pearled barley	¼ c	5	172
Scotch brand quick pearled barley	¼ c	5	172
Rice-A-Roni			
MICROWAVE LONG GRAIN & WILD RICE MIXES			
original flavor w/herbs & seasoning, prepared	½ c	840	140
chicken flavor & mushroom, prepared	½ c	720	140
RICE & PASTA MIXES			
beef flavor, prepared	1.33 oz	880	130
chicken & mushroom flavor, prepared	1.25 oz	790	130
chicken flavor & vegetables, prepared	1.2 oz	770	120
chicken flavor, prepared	1.33 oz	740	140
fried rice w/almonds, prepared	1.04 oz	670	110
herbs & butter, prepared	1.04 oz	760	110
rice pilaf, prepared	½ c	1,200	190
risotto, prepared	¾ c	1,110	210
Spanish rice, prepared	1.07 oz	950	110
Stroganoff w/sour cream sauce, prepared	1.35 oz	770	150
RICE MIXES			
brown & wild rice w/mushrooms, prepared	½ c	840	180
long grain & wild rice w/herbs & seasoning, prepared	½ c	630	140
yellow rice dinner, prepared	¾ c	1,160	250
River			
enriched rice	about ½ c cooked	<10	100
Success			
enriched, precooked, natural long grain rice	about ½ c cooked	0	100

	Portion	Sodium (mg)	Calories
Van Camp's			
Golden Hominy	1 c	701	128
Spanish rice	1 c	1,358	150
Water Maid			
enriched rice	about ½ c cooked	<10	100

❑ ROLLS *See* BREADS, ROLLS, BISCUITS, & MUFFINS

❑ SALAD DRESSINGS, MAYONNAISE, VINEGAR, & DIPS

Mayonnaise, Commercial

	Portion	Sodium (mg)	Calories
mayonnaise			
safflower & soybean	1 c	1,250	1,577
	1 T	79	99
soybean	1 c	1,250	1,577
	1 T	78	99
mayonnaise, imitation			
milk, cream	1 c	1,210	232
	1 T	76	15
soybean	1 c	1,193	556
	1 T	75	35
soybean w/out cholesterol	1 c	794	1,084
	1 T	49	68
mayonnaise-type dressing, regular	1 c	1,670	916
	1 T	104	57

Salad Dressings

	Portion	Sodium (mg)	Calories
bleu cheese, commercial, low-cal	1 T	155	11
coleslaw, commercial, low-cal	1 T	163	31
cooked, homemade	1 c	1,872	400
	1 T	117	25
French			
commercial			
regular	1 c	3,425	1,074
	1 T	214	67
creamy	1 T	125	70
low-cal	1 c	2,046	349
	1 T	128	22

	Portion	Sodium (mg)	Calories
homemade	1 c	1,448	1,388
	1 T	92	88
Green Goddess, commercial			
regular	1 T	150	68
low-cal	1 T	57	27
Italian, commercial			
regular	1 c	1,849	1,098
	1 T	116	69
creamy	1 T	105	52
low-cal	1 c	1,889	253
	1 T	118	16
Russian, commercial			
regular	1 c	2,127	1,210
	1 T	133	76
low-cal	1 c	2,257	368
	1 T	141	23
poppy seed	1 oz	271	121
sesame seed, commercial	1 c	2,450	1,086
	1 T	153	68
sweet & sour, commercial	1 T	68	29
Thousand Island, commercial			
regular	1 c	1,750	943
	1 T	109	59
low-cal	1 c	2,450	389
	1 T	153	24
vinegar & oil, homemade	1 c	1	1,122
	1 T	tr	72
vinegar (red wine) & oil, commercial	1 oz	423	103

Vinegar

	Portion	Sodium (mg)	Calories
cider	1 T	0	2
distilled	1 T	0	2

▪ BRAND NAME

Featherweight
LOW-SALT DRESSINGS

	Portion	Sodium (mg)	Calories
Soyamaise	1 T	3	100

LOW-SALT, LOW-CAL DRESSINGS

	Portion	Sodium (mg)	Calories
creamy cucumber	1 T	80	4
French	1 T	15	14
herb	1 T	5	6
Italian	1 T	120	4
New Bleu	1 T	110	4
red wine vinegar	1 T	100	6
Russian	1 T	125	6

	Portion	Sodium (mg)	Calories
Thousand Island	1 T	70	18
Zesty Tomato	1 T	5	2
Good Seasons Salad Dressing Mixes			
bleu cheese & herbs, w/vinegar, water, & salad oil	1 T	160	80
Buttermilk Farm Style, w/whole milk & mayonnaise	1 T	135	60
cheese garlic, w/vinegar, water, & salad oil	1 T	170	80
cheese Italian, w/vinegar, water, & salad oil	1 T	135	80
classic herb, w/vinegar, water, & salad oil	1 T	150	80
garlic & herbs, w/vinegar, water, & salad oil	1 T	190	80
Italian, w/vinegar, water, & salad oil	1 T	150	80
lemon & herbs, w/vinegar, water, & salad oil	1 T	140	80
lite Italian, w/vinegar, water, & salad oil	1 T	180	25
no-oil Italian, w/vinegar & water	1 T	30	6
Hellman's			
Light Reduced Calorie Mayonnaise	1 T	115	50
Real mayonnaise	1 T	80	100
sandwich spread	1 T	170	50
tartar sauce	1 T	220	70
Life All Natural			
avocado dressing/dip w/tofu	½ oz	75	70
creamy salad dressing, egg-free, low-cholesterol	½ oz	4	39
garlic dressing/dip w/tofu	½ oz	75	70
mayonnaise-style dressing, egg-free, low-cholesterol	½ oz	3	71
tofu dressing/dip	½ oz	75	75
Ortega			
Acapulco Dip	1 oz	0	8
Regina			
wine vinegars, all flavors	1 fl oz	0	4

❑ **SALADS, COMMERCIALLY PREPARED**
See FAST FOODS; FRUIT, FRESH
& PROCESSED; VEGETABLES, PLAIN
& PREPARED

	Portion	Sodium (mg)	Calories

❏ SAUCES, DESSERT *See* DESSERT SAUCES, SYRUPS, & TOPPINGS

❏ SAUCES, GRAVIES, & CONDIMENTS
See also FRUIT, FRESH & PROCESSED; PICKLES, OLIVES, RELISHES, & CHUTNEYS

Condiments

	Portion	Sodium (mg)	Calories
catsup	1 c	2,845	290
mustard, prepared, yellow	1 t	63	5

Gravies

	Portion	Sodium (mg)	Calories
au jus, dehydrated, prepared w/	1 c	579	19
water	21.7 oz	1,447	48
beef, canned	1 c	117	124
	10¼ oz	146	155
brown, dehydrated, prepared	1 c	125	9
w/water	9.7 oz	132	9
chicken			
canned	1 c	1,375	189
	10½ oz	1,718	236
dehydrated, prepared w/water	1 c	1,133	83
mushroom			
canned	1 c	1,359	120
	10½ oz	1,699	150
dehydrated, prepared w/water	1 c	1,402	70
onion, dehydrated, prepared w/water	1 c	1,036	80
pork, dehydrated, prepared w/water	1 c	1,235	76
turkey, dehydrated, prepared w/water	1 c	1,498	87

Sauces

	Portion	Sodium (mg)	Calories
béarnaise			
dehydrated	0.9 oz	841	90
dehydrated, prepared w/milk	1 c	1,265	701
& butter	13½ oz	1,897	1,052
barbecue, ready-to-serve	1 c	2,038	188

	Portion	Sodium (mg)	Calories
cheese			
dehydrated	1.2 oz	1,447	158
dehydrated, prepared w/whole milk	1 c	1,566	307
curry			
dehydrated	1.2 oz	1,444	151
dehydrated, prepared w/whole	1 c	1,276	270
milk	12 oz	1,595	337
hollandaise, dehydrated			
w/butterfat	1.2 oz	1,230	187
w/butterfat, prepared w/water	1 c	1,565	237
	7.2 oz	1,230	187
w/vegetable oil	1 oz	645	93
w/vegetable oil, prepared	1 c	1,134	703
w/milk & butter	13½ oz	1,701	1,055
marinara, canned	1 c	1,572	171
	15½ oz	2,760	300
mushroom			
dehydrated	1 oz	1,766	99
dehydrated, prepared w/whole	1 c	1,533	228
milk	11.7 oz	1,916	285
sour cream			
dehydrated	1.2 oz	444	180
dehydrated, prepared w/whole	1 c	1,007	509
milk	5½ oz	503	255
soy *See* SOYBEANS & SOYBEAN PRODUCTS			
spaghetti			
canned	1 c	1,236	272
	15½ oz	2,179	479
dehydrated	0.35 oz	848	28
	1½ oz	3,562	118
dehydrated, w/mushrooms	0.35 oz	942	30
	1.4 oz	3,674	118
Stroganoff			
dehydrated	1.6 oz	1,863	161
dehydrated, prepared w/whole	1 c	1,829	271
milk & water	11.2 oz	1,971	292
sweet & sour			
dehydrated	2 oz	584	220
dehydrated, prepared w/water	1 c	779	294
& vinegar	8.3 oz	584	220
tamari *See* SOYBEANS & SOYBEAN PRODUCTS			
teriyaki *See* SOYBEANS & SOYBEAN PRODUCTS			
tomato paste & puree *See* VEGETABLES, PLAIN & PREPARED			
tomato, canned	½ c	738	37
Spanish style	½ c	576	40

	Portion	Sodium (mg)	Calories
w/mushrooms	½ c	552	42
w/onions	½ c	672	52
w/tomato tidbits	½ c	18	39
white			
dehydrated	1.7 oz	1,691	230
dehydrated, prepared w/whole	1 c	796	241
milk	23.2 oz	1,990	602

▪ BRAND NAME

A-1
steak sauce	1 T	280	12

Chun King
mustard, brown	1 t	65	4
sauce/glaze mix for sweet & sour entree	3.8 oz	40	370
sweet & sour sauce	1.8 oz	240	60

Contadina Fresh Sauces
Alfredo	6 oz	020	540
Bolognese	7½ oz	600	230
Forestiera	7½ oz	830	270
marinara	7½ oz	700	100
pesto	3½ oz	540	510
plum tomato w/basil	7½ oz	700	100
red clam	7½ oz	800	120

Escoffier
Sauce Diable	1 T	160	20
Sauce Robert	1 T	70	20

Franco-American Gravies
au jus	2 oz	330	10
beef	2 oz	290	25
brown, w/onions	2 oz	340	25
chicken	2 oz	310	50
chicken giblet	2 oz	300	30
mushroom	2 oz	290	25
pork	2 oz	350	40
turkey	2 oz	290	30

Fresh Chef Sauces
Bolognese	4 oz	585	127
pesto	1 oz	244	155
red clam	4 oz	556	81
tomato	4 oz	686	151
white clam	4 oz	639	121

Grey Poupon
Dijon mustard	1 T	450	18

Health Valley
Catch-Up			
regular	1 T	190	16
no salt	1 T	70	16

	Portion	Sodium (mg)	Calories
tomato sauce			
regular	4 oz	460	70
no salt	4 oz	43	70
Life All Natural			
horseradish sauce	¼ fl oz	1	7
tartar sauce, egg-free, low-cholesterol	¼ fl oz	<2	19
tomato catsup	½ oz	4–9	17
Worcestershire sauce	¼ oz	2	5
Open Pit Barbecue Sauce			
original flavor	1 T	250	25
hickory smoke flavor	1 T	230	25
Hot 'n Tangy flavor	1 T	210	25
Mesquite 'n Tangy flavor	1 T	250	25
Sweet 'n Tangy flavor	1 T	190	25
Ortega			
enchilada sauce, mild or hot	1 oz	280	12
green chile salsa			
hot	1 oz	180	10
mild or medium	1 oz	180	8
Picante salsa	1 oz	300	10
Ranchera salsa	1 oz	250	12
taco salsa			
hot	1 oz	300	10
mild	1 oz	290	10
taco sauce			
hot	1 oz	210	12
mild	1 oz	220	12
Western-style taco sauce	1 oz	180	8
Prego			
Al Fresco Garden tomato sauce w/mushrooms or w/peppers	4 oz	560	100
Extra Chunky tomato sauce			
mushroom & green pepper	4 oz	440	110
mushroom & onion	4 oz	540	110
mushroom & tomato	4 oz	500	110
sausage & green pepper	4 oz	480	170
tomato & onion	4 oz	470	110
marinara sauce	4 oz	500	100
meat-flavored sauce	4 oz	630	150
mushroom tomato sauce	4 oz	630	140
no-salt-added tomato sauce	4 oz	25	100
regular tomato sauce	4 oz	630	140
Steak Supreme			
steak sauce	1 T	25	20
Wolf			
chili hot dog sauce	about ⅙ c	199	44

	Portion	Sodium (mg)	Calories

❏ SEAFOOD & SEAFOOD PRODUCTS
See also DINNERS, FROZEN;
ENTREES & MAIN COURSES, FROZEN

Finfish

ahi *See* tuna: yellowfin, *below*			
aku *See* tuna: skipjack, *below*			
anchovy, European			
raw	3 oz	88	111
canned in oil, drained solids	5	734	42
bass, freshwater			
mixed species, raw	3 oz	59	97
striped, raw	3 oz	59	82
bluefish, raw	3 oz	51	105
burbot, raw	3 oz	82	76
butterfish, raw	3 oz	75	124
carp			
raw	3 oz	42	108
baked, broiled, microwaved	3 oz	54	138
catfish			
channel			
raw	3 oz	54	99
breaded & fried	3 oz	238	194
ocean *See* wolffish, *below*			
chub *See* cisco: smoked, *below*			
cisco			
raw	3 oz	47	84
smoked	1 oz	135	50
	3 oz	409	151
cod			
Atlantic			
raw	3 oz	46	70
baked, broiled, microwaved	3 oz	66	89
canned, solids & liquids	3 oz	185	89
dried & salted	1 oz	1,968	81
	3 oz	5,973	246
Pacific, raw	3 oz	60	70
croaker, Atlantic			
raw	3 oz	47	89
breaded & fried	3 oz	296	188
cusk, raw	3 oz	27	74
dogfish *See* shark, *below*			
dolphin fish, raw	3 oz	74	73
drum, freshwater, raw	3 oz	64	101
eel, mixed species			
raw	3 oz	43	156
baked, broiled, microwaved	3 oz	55	200

	Portion	Sodium (mg)	Calories
flatfish			
raw	3 oz	69	78
baked, broiled, microwaved	3 oz	89	99
flounder *See* flatfish, *above*			
grouper, mixed species			
raw	3 oz	45	78
baked, broiled, microwaved	3 oz	45	100
haddock			
raw	3 oz	58	74
baked, broiled, microwaved	3 oz	74	95
smoked	1 oz	214	33
	3 oz	649	99
hake *See* whiting, *below*			
halibut			
Atlantic or Pacific			
raw	3 oz	46	93
baked, broiled, microwaved	3 oz	59	119
Greenland, raw	3 oz	68	158
herring			
Atlantic			
raw	3 oz	76	134
baked, broiled, microwaved	3 oz	98	172
canned *See* sardine: Atlantic, *below*			
kippered	1.4 oz	367	87
pickled	½ oz	131	39
lake *See* cisco, *above*			
Pacific, raw	3 oz	63	166
jack *See* mackerel: jack, *below*			
ling, raw	3 oz	115	74
lingcod, raw	3 oz	50	72
lox *See* salmon: chinook, smoked, *below*			
mackerel			
Atlantic			
raw	3 oz	76	174
baked, broiled, microwaved	3 oz	71	223
jack, canned, drained solids	1 c	720	296
king, raw	3 oz	134	89
Pacific & jack, mixed species, raw	3 oz	73	133
Spanish			
raw	3 oz	50	118
baked, broiled, microwaved	3 oz	56	134
mahimahi *See* dolphin fish, *above*			
monkfish, raw	3 oz	16	64
mullet, striped			
raw	3 oz	55	99
baked, broiled, microwaved	3 oz	61	127
ocean perch, Atlantic			
raw	3 oz	64	80
baked, broiled, microwaved	3 oz	82	103

	Portion	Sodium (mg)	Calories
perch, mixed species			
raw	3 oz	52	77
baked, broiled, microwaved	3 oz	67	99
pike			
northern			
raw	3 oz	33	75
baked, broiled, microwaved	3 oz	42	96
walleye, raw	3 oz	43	79
pollock			
Atlantic, raw	3 oz	73	78
walleye			
raw	3 oz	84	68
baked, broiled, microwaved	3 oz	98	96
pompano, Florida			
raw	3 oz	55	140
baked, broiled, microwaved	3 oz	65	179
porgy See scup, below			
pout, ocean, raw	3 oz	52	67
redfish See ocean perch, above			
rockfish, Pacific, mixed species			
raw	3 oz	51	80
baked, broiled, microwaved	3 oz	65	103
roughy, orange, raw	3 oz	54	107
sablefish			
raw	3 oz	48	166
smoked	1 oz	206	72
salmon			
Atlantic, raw	3 oz	37	121
chinook			
raw	3 oz	40	153
smoked	1 oz	220	33
	3 oz	666	99
chum			
raw	3 oz	42	102
canned, drained solids	3 oz	414	120
w/bone	13 oz	1,797	521
coho			
raw	3 oz	39	124
boiled, poached, steamed	3 oz	50	157
pink			
raw	3 oz	57	99
canned, solids w/bone & liq-	3 oz	471	118
uid	16 oz	2,514	631
red See salmon: sockeye, below			
sockey			
raw	3 oz	40	143
baked, broiled, microwaved	3 oz	56	183
canned, drained solids	3 oz	458	130
w/bone	13 oz	1,987	566

	Portion	Sodium (mg)	Calories
sardine			
Atlantic, canned in oil, drained solids w/bone	2 sardines = 0.8 oz	121	50
	3.2 oz	465	192
Pacific, canned in tomato sauce, drained solids w/ bone	1 sardine = 1.3 oz	157	68
	1.3 oz	1,532	658
	13 oz		
scrod *See* cod: Atlantic, *above*			
scup, raw	3 oz	36	89
sea bass, mixed species			
raw	3 oz	58	82
baked, broiled, microwaved	3 oz	74	105
sea trout, mixed species, raw	3 oz	49	88
shad, American, raw	3 oz	44	167
shark, mixed species			
raw	3 oz	67	111
batter-dipped & fried	3 oz	103	194
sheepshead			
raw	3 oz	61	92
baked, broiled, microwaved	3 oz	62	107
smelt, rainbow			
raw	3 oz	51	83
baked, broiled, microwaved	3 oz	65	106
snapper, mixed species			
raw	3 oz	54	85
baked, broiled, microwaved	3 oz	48	109
sole *See* flatfish, *above*			
spot, raw	3 oz	24	105
sturgeon, mixed species			
sucker, white, raw	3 oz	34	79
sunfish, pumpkinseed, raw	3 oz	68	76
swordfish			
raw	3 oz	76	103
baked, broiled, microwaved	3 oz	98	132
tilefish			
raw	3 oz	45	81
baked, broiled, microwaved	3 oz	50	125
trout			
mixed species, raw	3 oz	44	126
rainbow			
raw	3 oz	23	100
baked, broiled, microwaved	3 oz	29	129
tuna			
bluefin			
raw	3 oz	33	122
baked, broiled, microwaved	3 oz	43	157
light			
canned in soybean oil, drained solids	3 oz	301	169
	6 oz	606	339

	Portion	Sodium (mg)	Calories
canned in water, drained	3 oz	303	111
solids	5.8 oz	588	216
skipjack, raw	3 oz	31	88
white			
canned in soybean oil,	3 oz	336	158
drained solids	6.3 oz	704	331
canned in water, drained	3 oz	333	116
solids	6.1 oz	673	234
yellowfin, raw	3 oz	31	92
turbot			
domestic *See* halibut: Greenland, *above*			
European, raw	3 oz	127	81
whitefish, mixed species			
raw	3 oz	43	114
smoked	1 oz	285	30
	3 oz	866	92
whiting, mixed species			
raw	3 oz	61	77
baked, broiled, microwaved	3 oz	113	98
wolffish, Atlantic, raw	3 oz	72	82
yellowtail, mixed species, raw	3 oz	33	124

Shellfish

	Portion	Sodium (mg)	Calories
abalone, mixed species			
raw	3 oz	255	89
fried	3 oz	502	161
clams, mixed species			
raw	9 large (50/qt) or 20 small (110/qt)	100	133
	3 oz	47	63
boiled, poached, steamed	20 small (110/qt)	100	133
	3 oz	95	126
breaded & fried	20 small (110/qt)	684	379
	3 oz	309	171
canned, drained solids	3 oz	95	126
	1 c	179	236
canned, liquid	3 oz	183	2
	1 c	516	6
crab			
Alaska king			
raw	1 leg = 1 lb	1,438	144
	3 oz	711	71
boiled, poached, steamed	1 leg = 1 lb	1,436	129
	3 oz	911	82

	Portion	Sodium (mg)	Calories
crab *(cont.)*			
blue			
raw	1 crab = ⅓ lb	62	18
	3 oz	249	74
boiled, poached, steamed	3 oz	237	87
	1 c not packed	376	138
canned, dry pack or drained	3 oz	283	84
solids of wet pack	1 c not packed	450	133
Dungeness, raw	1 crab = 1½ lb	481	140
	3 oz	251	73
queen, raw	3 oz	458	76
crayfish, mixed species			
raw	3 oz	45	76
boiled, poached, steamed	3 oz	58	97
cuttlefish, mixed species, raw	3 oz	316	67
lobster, northern			
boiled, poached, steamed	3 oz	323	83
	1 c	551	142
mussels, blue			
raw	3 oz	243	73
	1 c	429	129
boiled, poached, steamed	3 oz	313	147
oysters			
eastern			
raw	6 medium (70/qt)	94	58
	1 c	277	170
breaded & fried	6 medium (70/qt)	367	173
	3 oz	355	167
boiled, poached, steamed	6 medium (70/qt)	94	58
	3 oz	190	117
canned, solids & liquids	3 oz	95	58
	1 c	277	170
Pacific, raw	1 medium (20/qt)	53	41
	3 oz	90	69
scallops, mixed species			
raw	2 large (30/lb) or 5 small (75/lb)	48	26
	3 oz	137	75
breaded & fried	2 large (30/lb)	144	67
shrimp, mixed species			
raw	4 large (32/lb)	42	30
	3 oz	126	90

	Portion	Sodium (mg)	Calories
boiled, poached, steamed	4 large (32/lb)	49	22
	3 oz	190	84
breaded & fried	4 large (32/lb)	103	73
	3 oz	292	206
canned, dry pack or drained	3 oz	143	102
solids of wet pack	1 c	216	154
snail, sea See whelk, *below*			
spiny lobster, mixed species, raw	1 lobster = 2 lb	370	233
	3 oz	150	95
squid, mixed species			
raw	3 oz	37	78
fried	3 oz	260	149
whelk			
raw	3 oz	175	117
boiled, poached, steamed	3 oz	350	233

Seafood Products

	Portion	Sodium (mg)	Calories
caviar, black & red, granular	1 T	240	40
	1 oz	420	71
crab cakes (blue crab)	2.1 oz	198	93
fish sticks (walleye pollock), frozen, reheated	1 stick = 1 oz	163	76
gefilte fish, commercial, sweet recipe w/broth	1½ oz	220	35
imitation seafood, made from surimi			
crab, Alaska king	3 oz	715	87
scallops, mixed species	3 oz	676	84
shrimp, mixed species	3 oz	599	86
surimi (processed from walleye pollock)	1 oz	40	28
	3 oz	122	84
tuna salad	3 oz	342	159
	1 c	824	383

▪ BRAND NAME

Featherweight

	Portion	Sodium (mg)	Calories
salmon, pink	2 oz	45	140
sardines			
canned in oil	1⅞ oz	65	130
canned in water	1⅞ oz	65	95
tuna, light chunk	2 oz	30	60

	Portion	Sodium (mg)	Calories
Fresh Chef			
seafood pasta salad	4.3 oz	426	229
Health Valley			
Best of Sea Food tuna	6 oz	754	160
No Salt Diet tuna	6 oz	106	160

❏ # SEASONINGS

See also BREADCRUMBS, CROUTONS, STUFFINGS, & SEASONED COATINGS; SAUCES, GRAVIES, & CONDIMENTS; VEGETABLES, PLAIN & PREPARED

	Portion	Sodium (mg)	Calories
allspice, ground	1 t	1	5
anise seed	1 t	tr	7
basil, ground	1 t	tr	4
bay leaf, crumbled	1 t	tr	2
caraway seed	1 t	tr	7
cardamon, ground	1 t	tr	6
celery seed	1 t	3	8
chervil, dried	1 t	tr	1
chili pepper	1 t	tr	9
chili powder	1 t	26	8
cinnamon sugar	1 t	0	16
cinnamon, ground	1 t	1	6
cloves, ground	1 t	5	7
coriander leaf, dried	1 t	1	2
coriander seed	1 t	1	5
cumin seed	1 t	4	8
curry powder	1 t	1	6
dill seed	1 t	tr	6
dillweed, dried	1 t	2	3
fennel seed	1 t	2	7
fenugreek seed	1 t	2	12
garlic powder	1 t	1	9
ginger, ground	1 t	1	6
mace, ground	1 t	1	8
marjoram, dried	1 t	tr	2
mustard powder	1 t	tr	9
mustard seed, yellow	1 t	tr	15
nutmeg, ground	1 t	tr	12
onion powder	1 t	1	7
oregano, ground	1 t	tr	5
paprika	1 t	1	6
parsley, dried	1 t	1	4
pepper, black	1 t	1	5
pepper, red/cayenne	1 t	1	6
pepper, seasoned	1 t	6	10

	Portion	Sodium (mg)	Calories
pepper, white	1 t	tr	7
poppy seed	1 t	tr	15
poultry seasoning	1 t	tr	5
pumpkin pie spice	1 t	1	6
rosemary, dried	1 t	1	4
saffron	1 t	1	2
sage, ground	1 t	tr	2
salt	1 t	2,300	0
savory, ground	1 t	tr	4
tarragon, ground	1 t	1	5
thyme, ground	1 t	1	4
tumeric, ground	1 t	1	8

▪ BRAND NAME

	Portion	Sodium (mg)	Calories
Diamond Crystal			
salt substitute	1 pkt	0	3
Featherweight			
salt substitute	¼ t	tr	0
seasoned salt substitute	¼ t	tr	0
French's			
imitation butter flavor salt	1 t	1,125	8
onion salt	1 t	1,590	6
seafood seasoning	1 t	1,410	2
seasoning salt	1 t	1,280	2
Kikkoman			
teriyaki baste & glaze	1 t	140	9
Lawry's			
onion salt	1 t	1,400	7
seasoning salt	1 t	1,164	3
McCormick's			
Season-All salt	1 t	980	4
Morton			
lite salt	1 t	1,100	0
salt substitute	1 t	0	0
Norcliff Thayer			
No Salt	1 pkt	0	0
Ortega			
mild taco meat seasoning	1 oz	1,970	90
Shake 'n Bake Seasoning Mixture			
Original Recipe			
for chicken	¼ pouch	450	80
for fish	¼ pouch	410	70
for pork	¼ pouch	600	80
for pork barbecue	¼ pouch	700	80
Country Mild recipe	¼ pouch	500	80
Italian herb recipe	¼ pouch	640	80

	Portion	Sodium (mg)	Calories

❑ SEEDS & SEED-BASED BUTTERS, FLOURS, & MEALS

See also NUTS & NUT-BASED BUTTERS, FLOURS, MEALS, MILKS, PASTES, & POWDERS

	Portion	Sodium (mg)	Calories
alfalfa seeds, sprouted, raw	1 c	2	10
cottonseed flour			
partially defatted	1 T	2	18
	1 c	33	337
low-fat	1 oz	10	94
cottonseed kernels, roasted	1 T	3	51
	1 c	37	754
cottonseed meal, partially defatted	1 oz	10	104
lotus seeds			
raw	1 oz	0	25
dried	1 oz	1	94
	1 c	1	106
pumpkin & squash seeds			
whole, roasted	1 oz	5	127
	1 c	12	285
kernels			
dried	1 oz	5	154
	1 c	24	747
roasted	1 oz	5	148
	1 c	40	1,184
sesame butter			
paste	1 T	2	95
	1 oz	3	169
tahini			
from raw & stone-ground	1 T	11	86
kernels	1 oz	21	162
from roasted & toasted	1 T	17	89
kernels	1 oz	33	169
from unroasted kernels	1 T	0	85
	1 oz	0	173
sesame flour			
high-fat	1 oz	12	149
partially defatted	1 oz	12	109
low-fat	1 oz	11	95
sesame meal, partially defatted	1 oz	11	161
sesame seeds			
whole			
dried	1 T	1	52
	1 c	16	825
roasted & toasted	1 oz	3	161

	Portion	Sodium (mg)	Calories
kernels			
dried	1 T	3	47
	1 c	59	882
toasted	1 oz	11	161
sisymbrium sp. seeds, whole,	1 oz	26	90
dried	1 c	68	235
squash seeds *See* pumpkin & squash seeds, *above*			
sunflower seed butter	1 T	1	93
sunflower seed flour, partially	1 T	0	16
defatted	1 c	2	261
sunflower seed kernels			
dried	1 oz	1	162
	1 c	4	821
dry-roasted	1 oz	1	165
	1 c	4	745
oil-roasted	1 oz	1	175
	1 c	4	830
toasted	1 oz	1	176
	1 c	4	829
tahini *See* sesame butter: tahini, *above*			
watermelon seed kernels, dried	1 oz	28	158
	1 c	107	602

▪ BRAND NAME

Arrowhead Mills
alfalfa seeds, sprouted	1 c	2	40
amaranth seeds	2 oz	2	200
flax seeds	1 oz	1	140
sesame seeds			
whole	1 oz	15	160
hulled	1 oz	9	160
sesame tahini, chemical-free	1 oz	2	170
sunflower seeds, hulled	1 oz	9	160

Planters
sunflower seeds	1 oz	30	160

❑ **SHERBETS** *See* DESSERTS, FROZEN

❑ **SHORTENINGS** *See* FATS, OILS, & SHORTENINGS

	Portion	Sodium (mg)	Calories

❑ SNACKS
See also CRACKERS

cheese puffs	1 oz	323	159
cheese straws	4	173	109
corn chips	1 oz	233	155
popcorn			
air-popped	1 c	tr	30
popped in vegetable oil	1 c	86	55
sugar-syrup-coated	1 c	tr	135
potato chips	10	94	105
made from dried potatoes	1 oz	216	164
potato sticks	1 oz	71	148
pretzels			
stick	10	48	10
twisted, Dutch	1	258	65
twisted, thin	10	966	240
tortilla chips	1 oz	155	150

▪ BRAND NAME

Arrowhead Mills

popcorn, unpopped	2 oz	2	210

Cornnuts

original flavor	1 oz	200	120
barbecue flavor	1 oz	290	110
nacho cheese flavor	1 oz	200	110
unsalted	1 oz	30	120

Del Monte

pineapple nuggets	0.9 oz	25	90
Sierra trail mix	0.9 oz	35	130
tropical fruit mix	0.9 oz	15	90
yogurt raisins			
plain	0.9 oz	25	120
strawberry	0.9 oz	20	120

Featherweight

cheese curls	1 oz	81	150
corn chips	1 oz	3	170
nacho cheese chips	1 oz	45	150
potato chips	1 oz	4	160
pretzels	3	5	20
round tortilla chips	1 oz	10	150

Health Valley
CORN CHIPS

regular	1 oz	90	163
no salt	1 oz	1	163
cheese corn chips, regular	1 oz	120	155

	Portion	Sodium (mg)	Calories
POTATO CHIPS			
Country Chips			
regular	1 oz	60	160
no salt	1 oz	1	160
Country Ripples			
regular	1 oz	60	160
no salt	1 oz	1	160
dip or regular	1 oz	60	160
no salt	1 oz	1	160
SNACK PUFFS			
Carrot Lites	1 oz	20	74
Cheddar Lites			
no salt	1 oz	70	60
w/green onion	1 oz	70	60
TORTILLA CHIPS			
Buenitos			
regular	1 oz	80	152
nacho cheese & CHILI	1 oz	60	150
no salt	1 oz	1	152
Mister Salty Pretzels			
butter-flavored sticks	90	620	110
Dutch	2	440	110
Junior	29	500	110
Mini Mix	23	480	110
sticks	90	620	110
Veri-Thin sticks	45	770	110
Nabisco			
DOO DADS			
Original	1 oz or ½ c	360	140
cheddar & herb	1 oz or ½ c	400	140
Zesty cheese	1 oz or ½ c	420	1t0
GREAT CRISPS!			
cheese & chive	9	170	70
French onion	7	90	70
Italian	9	200	70
nacho	8	250	70
Real bacon	9	230	70
savory garlic	8	190	70
sesame	9	190	70
sour cream & onion	8	200	70
tomato & celery	9	160	70
NIPS			
pizza	20	180	70
Real cheddar cheese	13	130	70
taco	14	200	70

	Portion	Sodium (mg)	Calories

Pepperidge Farm
SNACK STICKS

Original	8	320	130
cheese or sesame	8	340	130

TINY GOLDFISH

Original or cheddar cheese	45	180	140

Pillsbury Microwave Popcorn
FROZEN

original flavor	3 c popped	420	210
butter flavor	3 c popped	480	210
salt-free	3 c popped	0	170

SHELF-STABLE

original or butter flavor	3 c popped	410	210

Planters

Cheez Balls	1 oz	270	160
Cheez Curls	1 oz	290	160
corn chips	1 oz	160	160
Fruit 'n Nut Mix	1 oz	90	150
popcorn	3 c popped	0	20
microwave, butter or natural	3 c popped	560	140
Potato Crunchies	1¼ oz	310	190
pretzels	1 oz	700	110
round toast crackers	4	270	140
sour cream & onion puffs	1 oz	300	160
square cheese crackers	4	270	140

❑ SOUPS, PREPARED

Canned

asparagus, cream of, condensed	1 can = 10¾ oz	2,385	210
prepared w/water	1 c	981	87
prepared w/whole milk	1 c	1,041	161
	1 can	2,528	392
bean w/bacon, condensed	1 can = 11½ oz	2,311	420
prepared w/water	1 c	952	173
bean w/frankfurter, condensed	1 can = 11¼ oz	2,651	454
prepared w/water	1 c	1,092	187
bean w/ham, chunky, ready-to-serve	1 c	972	231
	1 can = 19¼ oz	2,184	519

	Portion	Sodium (mg)	Calories
bean, black, condensed	1 can = 11 oz	3,026	285
prepared w/water	1 c	1,198	116
beef broth or bouillon, ready-to-serve	1 c	782	16
	1 can = 14 oz	1,294	27
beef noodle, condensed	1 can = 10¾ oz	2,313	204
prepared w/water	1 c	952	84
beef, chunky, ready-to-serve	1 c	867	171
	1 can = 19 oz	1,947	383
celery, cream of, condensed	1 can = 10¾ oz	2,308	219
prepared w/water	1 c	942	90
prepared w/whole milk	1 c	1,010	165
	1 can	2,451	400
cheese, condensed	1 can = 11 oz	2,331	377
prepared w/water	1 c	959	155
prepared w/whole milk	1 c	1,020	230
	1 can	2,474	558
chicken & dumplings, condensed	1 can = 10½ oz	2,093	236
prepared w/water	1 c	861	97
chicken broth, condensed	1 can = 10¾ oz	1,909	94
prepared w/water	1 c	776	39
chicken gumbo, condensed	1 can = 10¾ oz	2,321	137
prepared w/water	1 c	955	56
chicken noodle, condensed	1 can = 10½ oz	2,257	182
prepared w/water	1 c	1,107	75
chicken noodle w/meatballs, ready-to-serve	1 c	1,039	99
	1 can = 20 oz	2,376	227
chicken rice			
chunky, ready-to-serve	1 c	888	127
	1 can = 19 oz	1,994	286
condensed	1 can = 10½ oz	1,980	146
prepared w/water	1 c	814	60
chicken vegetable			
chunky, ready-to-serve	1 c	1,068	167
	1 can = 19 oz	2,399	374
condensed	1 can = 10½ oz	2,297	181
prepared w/water	1 c	944	74
chicken, chunky, ready-to-serve	1 c	887	178
	1 can = 10¾ oz	1,078	216
chicken, cream of, condensed	1 can = 10¾ oz	2,397	283

	Portion	Sodium (mg)	Calories
chicken, cream of, condensed *(cont.)*			
prepared w/water	1 c	986	116
prepared w/whole milk	1 c	1,046	191
	1 can	2,540	464
chili beef, condensed	1 can = 11¼ oz	2,513	411
prepared w/water	1 c	1,035	169
clam chowder (Manhattan)			
chunky, ready-to-serve	1 c	1,000	133
	1 can = 19 oz	2,245	299
condensed	1 can = 10¾ oz	2,446	187
prepared w/water	1 c	1,808	78
clam chowder (New England), condensed	1 can = 10¾ oz	2,266	214
prepared w/water	1 c	914	95
prepared w/whole milk	1 c	992	163
	1 can	2,409	396
consommé w/gelatin, condensed	1 can = 10½ oz	1,550	71
prepared w/water	1 c	637	29
crab, ready-to-serve	1 c	1,234	76
	1 can = 13 oz	1,866	114
escarole, ready-to-serve	1 c	3,865	27
	1 can = 19½ oz	8,618	61
gazpacho, ready-to-serve	1 c	1,183	57
	1 can = 13 oz	1,790	87
lentil w/ham, ready-to-serve	1 c	1,318	140
	1 can = 20 oz	3,014	320
minestrone			
chunky, ready-to-serve	1 c	864	127
	1 can = 19 oz	1,940	285
condensed	1 can = 10½ oz	2,217	202
prepared w/water	1 c	911	83
mushroom w/beef stock, condensed	1 can = 10¾ oz	2,358	208
prepared w/water	1 c	970	85
mushroom, cream of, condensed	1 can = 10¾ oz	2,469	313
prepared w/water	1 c	1,031	129
prepared w/whole milk	1 c	1,076	203
	1 can	2,612	494
onion, condensed	1 can = 10½ oz	2,563	138
prepared w/water	1 c	1,053	57
oyster stew, condensed	1 can = 10½ oz	2,384	144
prepared w/water	1 c	980	59

	Portion	Sodium (mg)	Calories
prepared w/whole milk	1 c	1,040	134
	1 can	2,526	325
pea, green, condensed	1 can = 11¼ oz	2,397	398
prepared w/water	1 c	987	164
prepared w/whole milk	1 c	1,048	239
	1 can	2,541	579
pea, split, w/ham			
chunky, ready-to-serve	1 c	965	184
	1 can = 19 oz	2,167	413
condensed	1 can = 11½ oz	2,446	459
prepared w/water	1 c	1,008	189
pepperpot, condensed	1 can = 10½ oz	2,360	251
prepared w/water	1 c	970	103
potato, cream of, condensed	1 can = 10¾ oz	2,431	178
prepared w/water	1 c	1,000	73
prepared w/whole milk	1 c	1,060	148
	1 can	2,574	360
Scotch broth, condensed	1 can = 10½ oz	2,461	195
prepared w/water	1 c	1,012	80
shrimp, cream of, condensed	1 can = 10¾ oz	2,373	219
prepared w/water	1 c	970	90
prepared w/whole milk	1 c	1,036	165
	1 can	2,516	400
stockpot, condensed	1 can = 11 oz	2,546	242
prepared w/water	1 c	1,048	100
tomato beef w/noodle, condensed	1 can = 10¾ oz	2,230	341
prepared w/water	1 c	917	140
tomato bisque, condensed	1 can = 11 oz	2,546	300
prepared w/water	1 c	1,048	123
prepared w/whole milk	1 c	1,108	198
	1 can	2,689	481
tomato rice, condensed	1 can = 11 oz	1,981	291
prepared w/water	1 c	815	120
tomato, condensed	1 can = 10¾ oz	2,120	208
prepared w/water	1 c	872	86
prepared w/whole milk	1 c	932	160
	1 can	2,263	389
turkey noodle, condensed	1 can = 10¾ oz	1,983	168
prepared w/water	1 c	815	69
turkey vegetable, condensed	1 can = 10½ oz	2,202	179
prepared w/water	1 c	905	74

	Portion	Sodium (mg)	Calories
turkey, chunky, ready-to-serve	1 c	923	136
	1 can = 18¾ oz	2,082	306
vegetable w/beef broth, condensed	1 can = ½ oz	1,969	197
prepared w/water	1 c	810	81
vegetable w/beef, condensed	1 can = 10¾ oz	2,326	192
prepared w/water	1 c	957	79
vegetable, chunky, ready-to-serve	1 c	1,010	122
	1 can = 19 oz	2,269	274
vegetable, vegetarian, condensed	1 can = ½ oz	2,001	176
prepared w/water	1 c	823	72

Dehydrated

asparagus, cream of, prepared w/water	1 c	801	59
	39.7 oz	3,602	265
bean w/bacon, prepared w/water	1 c	928	105
beef broth or bouillon			
cubed	1 cube = 0.1 oz	864	6
prepared w/water	1 c	1,358	19
	6 fl oz	1,018	14
beef noodle, prepared w/water	1 c	1,041	41
	6 fl oz	775	30
cauliflower, prepared w/water	1 c	843	68
celery, cream of, prepared w/water	1 c	839	63
chicken broth or bouillon			
cubed	1 cube = 0.2 oz	1,152	9
prepared w/water	1 c	1,484	21
	6 fl oz	1,113	16
chicken noodle	1 pkt = 0.4 oz	931	38
	1 pkt = 2.6 oz	6,243	257
prepared w/water	1 c	1,284	53
chicken rice, prepared w/water	1 c	980	60
chicken vegetable, prepared w/water	1 c	808	49
	6 fl oz	606	37
chicken, cream of, prepared w/water	1 c	1,184	107
	6 fl oz	888	80
clam chowder (Manhattan)	1 c	1,336	65

	Portion	Sodium (mg)	Calories
clam chowder (New England)	1 c	745	95
consommé, w/gelatin added,	1 c	3,299	17
prepared w/water	39½ oz	14,853	77
leek, prepared w/water	1 c	966	71
	36 fl oz	4,345	319
minestrone, prepared w/water	1 c	1,026	79
	40.2 oz	4,618	358
mushroom	1 pkt instant = 0.6 oz	782	74
	1 pkt regular = 2.6 oz	3,482	328
prepared w/water	1 c	1,019	96
onion	1 pkt = ¼ oz	636	21
	1 pkt = 1.4 oz	3,493	115
prepared w/water	1 c	848	28
oxtail, prepared w/water	1 c	1,210	71
	36 fl oz	5,443	318
pea, green or split	1 pkt = 1 oz	914	100
	1 pkt = 4 oz	3,687	402
prepared w/water	1 c	1,220	133
tomato (includes cream of tomato)	1 pkt = ¾ oz	707	77
prepared w/water	1 c	943	102
	6 fl oz	708	77
tomato vegetable (includes Italian vegetable & spring vegetable)	1 pkt = 1.4 oz	2,588	125
prepared w/water	1 c	1,146	55
	6 fl oz	856	41
vegetable beef, prepared w/water	1 c	1,000	53
	1 pkt = 40 oz	4,513	240
vegetable, cream of, prepared w/water	1 c	1,171	105
	6 fl oz	878	79

▪ BRAND NAME

Campbell
CHUNKY SOUPS, READY-TO-SERVE

bean w/ham, Old Fashioned	11 oz	1,110	290
	9⅝ oz	960	260
beef	10¾ oz	1,090	190
	9½ oz	960	170
chicken, Old Fashioned	9½ oz	1,050	150
chicken mushroom, creamy	10½ oz	1,340	320
	9⅝ oz	1,200	280

	Portion	Sodium (mg)	Calories
chicken noodle	9½ oz	1,010	180
chicken noodle w/mushroom	10¾ oz	1,150	200
chicken rice	9½ oz	1,050	140
chicken vegetable	9½ oz	1,080	170
chili beef	11 oz	1,120	290
	9¾ oz	990	260
clam chowder (Manhattan style)	10¾ oz	1,230	160
	9½ oz	980	150
clam chowder (New England style)	10¾ oz	1,180	290
	9½ oz	1,040	250
Fisherman chowder	10¾ oz	1,290	260
	9½ oz	1,140	230
minestrone	9½ oz	890	160
mushroom, creamy	10½ oz	1,270	260
	9⅜ oz	1,130	240
sirloin burger	10¾ oz	1,240	220
	9½ oz	1,100	200
split pea & ham	10¾ oz	1,070	230
	9½ oz	950	210
steak & potato	10¾ oz	1,120	200
	9½ oz	990	170
Stroganoff-style beef	10¾ oz	1,230	300
turkey vegetable	9⅜ oz	1,060	150
vegetable	10¾ oz	1,100	140
	9½ oz	970	130
vegetable, Mediterranean	9½ oz	1,020	160
CONDENSED SOUPS, AS PACKAGED			
asparagus, cream of	4 oz	840	90
bean w/bacon	4 oz	850	150
beef broth (bouillon)	4 oz	820	16
beef noodle	4 oz	830	70
black bean	4 oz	950	110
celery, cream of	4 oz	830	100
cheddar cheese	4 oz	750	130
chicken & dumplings	4 oz	980	80
chicken broth	4 oz	750	35
chicken gumbo	4 oz	900	60
chicken noodle	4 oz	910	70
chicken vegetable	4 oz	850	70
chicken w/rice	4 oz	800	60
chicken, cream of	4 oz	810	110
chili beef	4 oz	740	130
clam chowder (Manhattan style)	4 oz	830	70
clam chowder (New England style)	4 oz	870	80
prepared w/whole milk	4 oz	930	150
French onion	4 oz	900	60
green pea	4 oz	830	160

	Portion	Sodium (mg)	Calories
minestrone	4 oz	910	80
mushroom, cream of	4 oz	820	100
mushroom, Golden	4 oz	870	80
nacho cheese	4 oz	750	100
noodles & ground beef	4 oz	830	90
onion, cream of	4 oz	830	100
prepared w/whole milk	4 oz	880	140
oyster stew	4 oz	830	80
prepared w/whole milk	4 oz	880	150
pepper pot	4 oz	960	90
potato, cream of	4 oz	880	70
prepared w/whole milk	4 oz	910	110
Scotch broth	4 oz	870	80
shrimp, cream of	4 oz	800	90
prepared w/whole milk	4 oz	850	160
split pea w/ham & bacon	4 oz	800	160
tomato	4 oz	670	90
prepared w/whole milk	4 oz	730	160
tomato bisque	4 oz	790	120
tomato rice, Old Fashioned	4 oz	730	110
turkey noodle	4 oz	870	70
turkey vegetable	4 oz	710	70
vegetable	4 oz	800	90
vegetable, Old Fashioned	4 oz	890	60
vegetable, vegetarian	4 oz	780	90
vegetable beef	4 oz	750	70
won ton	4 oz	870	40

CREAMY NATURAL SOUPS, CONDENSED

asparagus, prepared w/whole milk	4 oz	690	170
potato, prepared w/whole milk	4 oz	690	190

DRY SOUP MIXES, AS PACKAGED

chicken noodle	1 oz	810	100
chicken rice	1 oz	800	90
noodle	1 oz	760	110
onion	½ oz	730	50
onion mushroom	½ oz	740	50

HOME COOKIN' SOUPS, READY-TO-SERVE

chicken w/noodles	10¾ oz	1,130	140
country vegetable	10¾ oz	1,000	120
lentil	10¾ oz	940	170
minestrone	10¾ oz	1,210	140
split pea w/ham	10¾ oz	1,230	210
vegetable beef	10¾ oz	1,150	150

	Portion	Sodium (mg)	Calories
LOW-SODIUM SOUPS, READY-TO-SERVE			
chicken broth	10½ oz	70	40
chicken vegetable, chunky	10¾ oz	95	240
chicken w/noodles	10¾ oz	85	160
mushroom, cream of	10½ oz	60	200
split pea	10¾ oz	25	240
tomato w/tomato pieces	10½ oz	40	180
SEMICONDENSED SOUPS, AS PREPARED			
bean w/ham, Old Fashioned	11 oz	1,340	220
chicken & noodles, Golden	11 oz	1,450	120
clam chowder (New England)	11 oz	1,360	130
prepared w/whole milk	11 oz	1,410	190
mushroom, savory cream of	11 oz	1,500	180
Tomato Royale	11 oz	1,290	180
vegetable, Old World	11 oz	1,470	130
College Inn			
beef broth	1 c	1,280	18
chicken broth	1 c	1,320	35
Featherweight			
bouillon, instant			
beef	1 t	10	18
chicken	1 t	5	18
chicken noodle	7½ oz	405	80
mushroom	7½ oz	320	60
tomato	7½ oz	240	70
vegetable beef	7½ oz	300	100
Health Valley			
bean			
regular	7½ oz	430	154
no salt	7½ oz	20	154
five bean, chunky			
regular	7½ oz	480	100
no salt	7½ oz	60	100
beef broth			
regular	7½ oz	420	8
no salt	7½ oz	5	8
chicken broth, regular	7½ oz	410	34
clam chowder			
regular	7½ oz	470	110
no salt	7½ oz	60	110
green split pea			
regular	7½ oz	440	158
no salt	7½ oz	25	158
lentil			
regular	7½ oz	440	163
no salt	7½ oz	25	163

	Portion	Sodium (mg)	Calories
minestrone			
regular	7½ oz	490	115
no salt	7½ oz	80	115
mushroom barley			
regular	7½ oz	440	107
no salt	7½ oz	20	110
potato leek			
regular	7½ oz	430	107
no salt	7½ oz	20	107
tomato			
regular	7½ oz	450	100
no salt	7½ oz	40	100
vegetable			
regular	7½ oz	460	100
no salt	7½ oz	40	100
vegetable chicken, chunky			
regular	7½ oz	448	217
no salt	7½ oz	56	217
Nissin			
CUP O'NOODLES			
beef	1 pkg = 1 c	1,490	290
chicken	1 pkg = 1 c	1,790	300
shrimp	1 pkg = 1 c	1,480	300
HEARTY CUP O'NOODLES			
cream of chicken	1 pkg = 1 c	1,450	300
OODLES OF NOODLES			
beef	1 pkg = 1 c	1,910	390
chicken	1 pkg = 1 c	1,660	400
TWIN CUP O'NOODLES			
chicken	1 pkg = 1 c	910	150
Rokeach Condensed Soups			
barley & mushroom	8 fl oz	904	85
celery, cream of			
prepared w/water	5 oz	950	90
prepared w/milk	5 oz	1,020	190
mushroom, cream of			
prepared w/water	5 oz	1,050	150
prepared w/milk	5 oz	1,170	240
split pea or egg & barley	8 fl oz	757	132
tomato			
prepared w/water	5 oz	980	90
prepared w/milk	5 oz	1,054	190
tomato w/rice	5 oz	815	160
vegetarian vegetable	5 oz	1,055	90
Swanson			
beef broth	7¼ oz	750	20
chicken broth	7¼ oz	910	30

	Portion	Sodium (mg)	Calories

❑ **SOUR CREAM** *See* **MILK, MILK SUBSTITUTES, & MILK PRODUCTS**

❑ **SOYBEANS & SOYBEAN PRODUCTS**

Soybeans

boiled	½ c	1	149
dry-roasted	½ c	2	387
mature seeds, sprouted, steamed	½ c	5	38
roasted	½ c	140	405

Soybean Products

fermented products			
miso	½ c	5,032	284
natto	½ c	6	187
tempeh	½ c	5	165
soy flour			
full-fat			
raw	½ c stirred	5	182
roasted	½ c stirred	5	184
low-fat	½ c stirred	8	163
defatted	½ c stirred	10	164
soy meal, defatted, raw	½ c	2	206
soy milk, fluid	1 c	30	79
soy protein			
concentrate	1 oz	1	92
isolate	1 oz	281	94
soy sauce			
made from hydrolyzed vegetable protein	1 T	1,024	7
	¼ c	3,300	24
made from soy (tamari)	1 T	1,005	11
	¼ c	3,240	35
made from soy & wheat (shoyu)	1 T	1,029	9
	¼ c	3,314	30
teriyaki sauce			
dehydrated	1 pkt = 1.6 oz	4,784	130
prepared w/water	1 c	4,791	131
ready-to-serve	1 T	690	15
	1 fl oz	1,380	30
tofu			
dried-frozen (koyadofu)			
prepared w/nigari	0.6 oz	1	82
prepared w/calcium sulfate	0.6 oz	1	82

	Portion	Sodium (mg)	Calories
fried			
prepared w/calcium sulfate	½ oz	2	35
prepared w/nigari	½ oz	2	35
okara	½ c	6	47
raw			
regular, made w/nigari	4.1 oz	8	88
	½ c	9	94
regular, made w/calcium sulfate	4.1 oz	8	88
	½ c	9	94
firm, made w/nigari	2.9 oz	192	118
	½ c	298	183
firm, made w/calcium sulfate	2.9 oz	192	118
	½ c	298	183
salted & fermented (fuyu)			
prepared w/nigari	0.4 oz	316	13
prepared w/calcium sulfate	0.4 oz	310	13

▪ BRAND NAME

Arrowhead Mills

soy flour	2 oz	1	250
soybean flakes	2 oz	3	250
soybeans	2 oz	3	230
tamari soy sauce	1 T	800	15

Chun King

soy sauce	1 t	430	6

Fearn

lecithin granules	2 level T	5	100
liquid lecithin			
regular	1 T	0	130
mint-flavored	1 T	0	113
natural soya powder	¼ c	<5	100
soya granules	¼ c	5	140
soya protein isolate	¼ c	130	60

Health Valley

Soy Moo soybean milk	8 fl oz	55	125

Kikkoman

soy sauce			
regular	1 T	892	10
lite	1 T	600	11
stir-fry sauce	1 t	120	6
sweet & sour sauce	1 T	63	18
teriyaki sauce	1 T	630	15

❑ SPICES *See* SEASONINGS

	Portion	Sodium (mg)	Calories

❑ **STUFFINGS** *See* BREADCRUMBS, CROUTONS, STUFFINGS, & SEASONED COATINGS

❑ **SUGARS & SWEETENERS: HONEY, MOLASSES, SUGAR, SUGAR SUBSTITUTES, SYRUP, & TREACLE**

	Portion	Sodium (mg)	Calories
HONEY			
honey	1 T	1	64
	5 T	5	320
MOLASSES			
first extraction, light	1 T	16	50
	5 T	80	252
SUGAR			
brown	1 T	3	52
	5 T	17	364
white			
granulated	1 t	0	16
	1 T	0	46
	½ c	2	335
powdered	1 c	1	462
SYRUP			
corn	1 T	14	59
	5 T	70	295
dark corn	1 T	40	60
maple	1 T	2	50
	5 T	10	252
maple, imitation	1 T	35	55
	5 T	175	275
table blend, pancake			
mainly corn	1 T	13	57
	5 T	68	286
cane & maple	1 T	tr	50
TREACLE			
black	1 T	19	53
	5 T	96	265

	Portion	Sodium (mg)	Calories
▪ **BRAND NAME**			
Aunt Jemima			
Butter Lite syrup	1 fl oz	67	52
Lite syrup	1 fl oz	66	60
syrup	1 fl oz	21	103
Brer Rabbit			
molasses			
dark	1 T	15	60
light	1 T	10	60
Diamond Crystal			
sugar substitute	1 pkg	tr	1
Golden Griddle			
syrup	1 T	15	50
Grandma's Molasses			
gold label	1 T	28	70
green label	1 T	57	70
Karo			
corn syrup			
dark	1 T	40	60
light	1 T	30	60
pancake syrup	1 T	35	60
Log Cabin			
buttered syrup	1 fl oz	74	105
Country Kitchen syrup	1 fl oz	19	101
maple honey syrup	1 fl oz	7	106
syrup	1 fl oz	38	99
Sprinkle Sweet			
sugar substitute	⅛ t	1	2
Sugartwin			
sugar substitute			
white	1 pkg	2	3
white/brown	1 t	2	1
Sweet & Low			
sugar substitute	1 pkg	4	4
Sweet 10			
sugar substitute	⅛ t	0	0
Vermont Maid			
syrup	1 T	5	50

	Portion	Sodium (mg)	Calories

❏ **SYRUP** *See* SUGARS & SWEETENERS

❏ **SYRUP, DESSERT** *See* DESSERT SAUCES, SYRUPS, & TOPPINGS

❏ **TOFU, FROZEN** *See* DESSERTS, FROZEN

❏ **TREACLE** *See* SUGARS & SWEETENERS

❏ **TURKEY** *See* POULTRY, FRESH & PROCESSED; PROCESSED MEAT & POULTRY PRODUCTS

❏ **VEAL** *See* LAMB, VEAL, & MISCELLANEOUS MEATS

❏ **VEGETABLES, PLAIN & PREPARED**
See also LEGUMES & LEGUME PRODUCTS; PICKLES, OLIVES, RELISHES, & CHUTNEYS; RICE & GRAINS, PLAIN & PREPARED

Vegetables, Plain

	Portion	Sodium (mg)	Calories
alfalfa seeds *See* SEEDS & SEED-BASED BUTTERS, FLOURS, & MEALS			
amaranth			
raw	1 c	5	7
boiled, drained	½ c	14	14
arrowhead			
raw	1 medium corm = 0.4 oz	3	12
boiled, drained	1 medium corm = 1.4 oz	2	9
artichokes, globe & French varieties			
boiled	1 medium = 4.2 oz	79	53
	½ c hearts	55	37

	Portion	Sodium (mg)	Calories
frozen, boiled, drained	9 oz pkg	127	108
asparagus beans *See* yardlong beans, *under* LEGUMES & LEGUME PRODUCTS			
asparagus, cuts & spears			
raw	4 spears = 2 oz	1	13
boiled	4 spears = 2.1 oz	3	15
canned, solids & liquids	½ c	425	17
frozen, boiled, drained	4 spears = 2.1 oz	2	17
	10 oz pkg	12	82
balsam pear			
leafy tips			
raw	½ c	3	7
boiled, drained	½ c	4	10
pods			
raw	1 c	5	16
boiled, drained	½ c	4	12
bamboo shoots			
raw	½ c	3	21
boiled, drained	1 c	5	15
canned, drained solids	1 c	9	25
beans, shellie, canned, solids & liquids	½ c	408	37
beans, snap			
raw	½ c	3	17
boiled, drained	½ c	2	22
canned			
drained solids	½ c	170	13
solids & liquids	½ c	442	18
solids & liquids, seasoned	½ c	425	18
frozen, boiled, drained	½ c	9	18
beet greens			
raw	½ c	38	4
boiled, drained	½ c	42	20
beets			
raw	½ c sliced	49	30
boiled, drained	½ c sliced	173	26
canned, solids & liquids	½ c sliced	324	36
pickled, canned, solids & liquids	½ c	301	75
beets, Harvard, canned, solids & liquids	½ c sliced	199	89
bittergourd; bittermelon *See* balsam pear, *above*			
bok choy *See* cabbage, Chinese, *below*			
borage			
raw	½ c	35	9
boiled, drained	3½ oz	88	25
broad beans *See* LEGUMES & LEGUME PRODUCTS			

	Portion	Sodium (mg)	Calories
broccoli			
raw	1 spear = 5.3 oz	40	42
boiled, drained	1 spear = 6.3 oz	19	53
	½ c	8	23
frozen, boiled, drained	½ c chopped	22	25
	½ c spears	60	69
	10 oz pkg spears	22	25
brussels sprouts			
boiled, drained	1 sprout = 0.73 oz	4	8
	½ c	17	30
frozen, boiled, drained	½ c	18	33
burdock root			
raw	1 c	6	85
	5½ oz	8	112
boiled, drained	1 c	5	110
	5.8 oz	7	146
butterbur			
raw	1 c	7	13
boiled, drained	3½ oz	4	8
cabbage			
raw	½ c shredded	6	8
boiled, drained	½ c shredded	14	16
cabbage, Chinese			
bok choy			
raw	½ c shredded	23	5
boiled, drained	½ c shredded	29	10
pe-tsai			
raw	½ c shredded	3	6
boiled, drained	1 c shredded	11	16
cabbage, red			
raw	½ c shredded	4	10
boiled, drained	½ c shredded	6	16
cabbage, savoy			
raw	½ c shredded	10	10
boiled, drained	½ c shredded	17	18
cardoon, raw	½ c shredded	151	18
carrots			
raw	½ c shredded	19	24
	2½ oz	25	31
boiled, drained	½ c sliced	52	35
	1.6 oz	30	21
canned			
drained solids	½ c sliced	176	17
solids & liquids	½ c sliced	297	28
frozen, boiled, drained	½ c sliced	43	26
cassava, raw	3½ oz	8	120

	Portion	Sodium (mg)	Calories
cauliflower			
raw	3 flowerets = 2 oz	8	13
	½ c pieces	7	12
boiled, drained	½ c pieces	4	15
frozen, boiled, drained	½ c pieces	16	17
celeriac			
raw	½ c	78	31
boiled, drained	3½ oz	61	25
celery			
raw	½ c diced	53	9
	1 stalk = 1.4 oz	35	6
boiled, drained	½ c diced	48	11
celtuce, raw	1 leaf = 0.3 oz	1	2
chard, Swiss			
raw	½ c chopped	38	3
boiled, drained	½ c chopped	158	18
chayote, fruit			
raw	1 c pieces	5	32
	7.1 oz	8	49
boiled, drained	1 c pieces	1	38
chicory, raw			
greens	½ c chopped	41	21
roots	½ c pieces	23	33
witloof	½ c	3	7
Chinese parsley See coriander, below			
Chinese preserving melon See wax gourd, below			
chives, raw	1 t	0	0
	1 T	0	1
chrysanthemum, garland			
raw	1 c pieces	13	4
boiled, drained	½ c pieces	27	10
collards			
raw	½ c chopped	26	18
boiled, drained	½ c chopped	18	13
frozen, boiled, drained	½ c chopped	42	31
coriander (cilantro), raw	¼ c	1	1
corn, sweet			
raw	kernels from 1 ear	14	77
	½ c kernels	12	66
boiled, drained	½ c kernels	14	89
	kernels from 1 ear	13	83
canned			
cream style	½ c	365	93
in brine, solids & liquids	½ c	324	79
w/red & green peppers, solids & liquids	½ c	396	86

	Portion	Sodium (mg)	Calories
corn, sweet: canned *(cont.)*			
vacuum pack	½ c	286	83
frozen, boiled, drained	½ c kernels	4	67
	kernels from 1 ear	3	59
cowpeas *See* LEGUMES & LEGUME PRODUCTS			
cress, garden			
raw	1 sprig	0	0
	½ c	4	8
boiled, drained	½ c	5	16
cucumber, raw	½ c sliced	1	7
	10½ oz	6	39
daikon *See* radishes: Oriental, *below*			
dandelion greens			
raw	½ c chopped	21	13
boiled, drained	½ c chopped	23	17
dasheen *See* taro, *below*			
dock			
raw	½ c chopped	3	15
boiled, drained	3½ oz	3	20
eggplant, boiled, drained	1 c cubed	2	27
endive, Belgian *See* chickory: witloof, *above*			
endive, raw	½ c chopped	6	4
eppaw, raw	½ c	6	75
escarole *See* endive, *above*			
garlic, raw	1 clove = 0.1 oz	1	4
ginger root, raw	0.4 oz	1	8
	¼ c sliced	3	17
gourd			
dishcloth, boiled, drained	½ c sliced	18	50
white-flowered (calabash), boiled, drained	½ c cubed	1	11
horseradish-tree			
leafy tips			
raw	½ c chopped	1	6
boiled, drained	½ c chopped	2	13
pods			
raw	1 pod = 0.4 oz	5	4
boiled, drained	½ c sliced	25	21
hyacinth beans *See* LEGUMES & LEGUME PRODUCTS			
jicama *See* yam bean, *below*			
jute (pot herb), boiled, drained	½ c	5	16
kale			
raw	½ c chopped	15	17
boiled, drained	½ c chopped	15	21
frozen, boiled, drained	½ c chopped	10	20
kale, Scotch			
raw	½ c chopped	24	14
boiled, drained	½ c chopped	29	18

	Portion	Sodium (mg)	Calories
kanpyo (dried gourd strips)	0.7 oz	3	49
kohlrabi			
raw	½ c sliced	14	19
boiled, drained	½ c sliced	17	24
leeks			
raw	¼ c chopped	5	16
boiled, drained	¼ c chopped	3	8
freeze-dried	1 T	0	1
lentils *See* LEGUMES & LEGUME PRODUCTS			
lettuce, raw			
butterhead (includes Boston & Bibb types)	2 leaves = ½ oz	1	2
	1 head = 5.7 oz	8	21
cos or romaine	1 inner leaf = 0.35 oz	1	2
	½ c shredded	2	4
iceberg	1 leaf = 0.7 oz	2	3
	1 head = 1 lb 3 oz	48	70
looseleaf	1 leaf = 0.35 oz	1	2
	½ c shredded	3	5
lima beans *See* LEGUMES & LEGUME PRODUCTS			
lotus root, boiled, drained	3.1 oz	40	59
manioc *See* cassava, *above*			
mountain yam, Hawaii, steamed	½ c	9	59
mung beans *See* LEGUMES & LEGUME PRODUCTS			
mushrooms			
raw	½ c pieces	1	9
boiled, drained	½ c pieces	2	21
mushrooms, shitake			
cooked	½ oz	3	40
dried	0.1 oz	0	11
mustard greens			
raw	½ c chopped	7	7
boiled, drained	½ c chopped	11	11
frozen, boiled, drained	½ c chopped	19	14
New Zealand spinach			
raw	½ c chopped	36	4
boiled, drained	½ c chopped	97	11
okra			
boiled, drained	½ c sliced	4	25
frozen, boiled, drained	½ c sliced	3	34
onions			
raw	1 T chopped	0	3
	½ c chopped	2	27
boiled, drained	1 T chopped	1	4
	½ c chopped	8	29

	Portion	Sodium (mg)	Calories
onions *(cont.)*			
canned, solids & liquids	2.2 oz	234	12
dehydrated flakes	1 T	1	16
frozen, boiled, drained	1 T chopped	2	4
	½ c chopped	13	30
onions, spring, raw	1 T chopped	0	2
	½ c chopped	2	13
oysterplant *See* salsify, *below*			
parsley			
raw	10 sprigs = 0.35 oz	4	3
	½ c chopped	12	10
freeze-dried	1 T	2	1
parsnips			
raw	½ c sliced	7	50
boiled, drained	½ c sliced	8	63
peas & carrots			
canned, solids & liquids	½ c	332	48
frozen, boiled, drained	½ c	55	38
	10 oz pkg	190	133
peas & onions, canned, solids & liquids	½ c	265	30
peas, edible pods			
raw	½ c	3	30
boiled, drained	½ c	3	34
frozen, boiled, drained	½ c	4	42
	10 oz pkg	12	132
peas, green			
raw	½ c	4	63
boiled, drained	½ c	2	67
canned			
drained solids	½ c	186	59
solids & liquids	½ c	340	61
solids & liquids, seasoned	½ c	290	57
frozen, boiled, drained	½ c	70	63
peas, mature seeds, sprouted			
raw	½ c	12	77
boiled, drained	3½ oz	3	118
peas, split *See* split peas, *under* LEGUMES & LEGUME PRODUCTS			
pepeao			
raw	0.2 oz	1	2
dried	½ c	8	36
peppers			
hot chili			
raw	1 pepper = 1.6 oz	3	18
	½ c chopped	5	30

	Portion	Sodium (mg)	Calories
jalapeño, canned, solids & liquids	½ c chopped	995	17
sweet			
raw	1 pepper = 2.6 oz	2	18
	½ c chopped	2	12
boiled, drained	1 pepper = 2.6 oz	2	13
	½ c chopped	1	12
canned, solids & liquids	½ c halves	958	13
freeze-dried	1 T	1	1
	¼ c	3	5
frozen, unprepared, chopped	10 oz pkg	15	58
frozen, boiled, drained	3½ oz chopped	4	18
pigeon peas *See* LEGUMES & LEGUME PRODUCTS			
pimientos *See* PICKLES, OLIVES, RELISHES, & CHUTNEYS			
pinto beans *See* LEGUMES & LEGUME PRODUCTS			
poi	½ c	14	134
potatoes			
raw			
flesh	3.9 oz	7	88
skin	1.3 oz	4	22
baked			
flesh & skin	7.1 oz	16	220
flesh	5½ oz	8	145
skin	2 oz	12	115
boiled n skin			
flesh	4.8 oz	6	119
skin	1.2 oz	5	27
boiled w/out skin, flesh	4.8 oz	7	116
canned, solids & liquids	1 c	904	120
frozen, whole, unprepared	½ c	22	71
microwaved in skin			
flesh & skin	7.1 oz	16	212
flesh	5½ oz	11	156
skin	2 oz	9	77
pumpkin			
boiled, drained	½ c mashed	2	24
canned	½ c	6	41
pumpkin flowers			
raw	1 c	2	5
boiled, drained	½ c	4	10
pumpkin leaves, boiled, drained	½ c	3	7
purslane			
raw	1 c	51	7
boiled, drained	1 c	20	21
radish seeds, sprouted, raw	½ c	1	8
radishes, raw	10 radishes = 1.6 oz	11	7

	Portion	Sodium (mg)	Calories
radishes, raw *(cont.)*			
Oriental			
raw	½ c	9	8
boiled, drained	½ c sliced	10	13
dried	½ c	161	157
white icicle, raw	½ c sliced	8	7
rutabagas			
raw	½ c cubed	14	25
boiled, drained	½ c mashed	22	41
	½ c cubed	15	29
salsify			
raw	½ c sliced	13	55
boiled, drained	½ c sliced	11	46
seaweed			
agar, raw	3½ oz	9	26
kelp, raw	3½ oz	233	43
laver, raw	3½ oz	48	35
spirulina			
raw	3½ oz	98	26
dried	3½ oz	1,048	290
wakame, raw	3½ oz	872	45
sesbania flower			
raw	1 c	3	5
steamed	1 c	11	23
shallots			
raw	1 T chopped	1	7
freeze-dried	1 T	1	3
snow peas *See* peas, edible pods, *above*			
soybeans *See* SOYBEANS & SOYBEAN PRODUCTS			
spinach			
raw	½ c chopped	22	6
boiled, drained	½ c	63	21
canned			
drained solids	½ c	29	25
solids & liquids	½ c	373	22
frozen, boiled, drained	½ c	82	27
	10 oz pkg	190	63
spinach, New Zealand *See* New Zealand spinach, *above*			
split peas *See* LEGUMES & LEGUME PRODUCTS			
sprouts *See plant name (alfalfa, mung bean, etc.)*			
squash, summer			
crookneck			
raw	½ c sliced	1	12
canned, drained solids	½ c sliced	5	14
boiled, drained	½ c sliced	1	18
frozen, boiled, drained	½ c sliced	6	24
scallop			
raw	½ c sliced	1	12
boiled, drained	½ c sliced	1	14
zucchini			
raw	½ c sliced	2	9

	Portion	Sodium (mg)	Calories
boiled, drained	½ c sliced	2	14
canned, Italian style, in tomato sauce	½ c	427	33
frozen, boiled, drained	½ c	2	19
other varieties			
raw	½ c sliced	1	13
boiled, drained	½ c sliced	1	18
squash, winter			
acorn			
baked	½ c cubed	4	57
boiled	½ c mashed	3	41
butternut			
baked	½ c cubed	4	41
frozen, boiled	½ c mashed	2	47
hubbard			
baked	½ c cubed	8	51
boiled	½ c mashed	6	35
spaghetti, boiled, drained, baked	½ c	14	23
other varieties			
raw	½ c cubed	2	21
baked	½ c cubed	1	39
string beans See beans, snap, above			
succotash			
boiled, drained	½ c	16	111
canned			
w/cream-style corn	½ c	325	102
w/whole kernel corn, solids & liquids	½ c	283	81
frozen, boiled, drained	½ c	38	79
swamp cabbage			
raw	1 c chopped	63	11
boiled, drained	1 c chopped	119	20
sweet potato leaves			
raw	1 c chopped	3	12
steamed	1 c	8	22
sweet potatoes			
baked in skin	1 potato = 4 oz	12	118
	½ c mashed	10	103
boiled w/out skin	½ c mashed	21	172
candied	3.7 oz	73	144
canned			
mashed	1 c	191	258
in syrup, drained solids	1 c	76	213
in syrup, solids & liquids	1 c	100	202
vacuum packed	1 c pieces	107	183
	1 c mashed	136	233
frozen, baked	½ c cubed	7	88
Swiss chard See chard, Swiss, above			

	Portion	Sodium (mg)	Calories
taro			
raw	½ c sliced	6	56
cooked	½ c sliced	10	94
taro chips	10 chips = 0.8 oz	85	110
taro leaves			
raw	1 c	1	12
steamed	1 c	3	35
taro shoots			
raw	1 shoot = 2.9 oz	1	9
cooked	½ c sliced	1	10
taro, Tahitian			
raw	½ c sliced	31	25
cooked	½ c sliced	37	30
tomatoes, green, raw	1 tomato = 4.3 oz	16	30
tomatoes, red, ripe			
raw	1 tomato = 4.3 oz	10	24
boiled	½ c	13	30
canned			
whole	½ c	195	24
stewed	½ c	325	34
wedges in juice	½ c	285	34
w/green chilies	½ c	481	18
stewed	1 c	374	59
tomato paste, canned	½ c	86	110
tomato puree, canned	1 c	49	102
tomato sauce See SAUCES, GRAVIES, & CONDIMENTS			
towel gourd See gourd: dishcloth, above			
tree fern, cooked	½ c chopped	3	28
turnip greens			
raw	½ c chopped	11	7
boiled, drained	½ c chopped	21	15
canned, solids & liquids	½ c	325	17
frozen, boiled, drained	½ c	12	24
turnip greens & turnips, frozen, boiled, drained	3½ oz	15	17
turnips			
raw	½ c cubed	44	18
boiled, drained	½ c cubed	39	14
frozen, boiled, drained	3½ oz	36	23
vegetables, mixed			
canned			
drained solids	½ c	122	39
solids & liquids	½ c	273	44
frozen, boiled, drained	½ c	32	54
	10 oz pkg	96	163

	Portion	Sodium (mg)	Calories
water chestnuts, Chinese			
raw	1¼ oz	5	38
canned, solids & liquids	1 oz	2	14
watercress, raw	½ c chopped	7	2
wax beans *See* beans, snap, *above*			
wax gourd (Chinese preserving melon), boiled, drained	½ c cubed	93	11
winged beans *See* LEGUMES & LEGUME PRODUCTS			
yam, baked or boiled	½ c cubed	6	79
yam bean (tuber only)			
raw	1 c sliced	8	49
boiled, drained	3½ oz	6	46
yardlong beans *See* LEGUMES & LEGUME PRODUCTS			

Vegetables, Prepared

	Portion	Sodium (mg)	Calories
coleslaw	½ c	14	42
corn pudding	1 c	138	271
onion rings, breaded, frozen, heated in oven	0.7 oz	75	81
potatoes, au gratin			
dry mix, prepared	5½ oz pkg	3,609	764
homemade	½ c	528	160
potatoes, french fried, frozen			
cottage-cut, heated in oven	1.8 oz	23	109
extruded, heated in oven	1.8 oz	307	163
fried in animal fat & vegetable oil	1.8 oz	108	158
fried in vegetable oil	1.8 oz	108	158
heated in oven	1.8 oz	15	111
potatoes, hashed brown			
frozen, plain, prepared	½ c	27	170
frozen, w/butter sauce, unprepared	6 oz pkg	130	229
homemade, prepared in vegetable oil	½ c	19	163
potatoes, mashed			
dehydrated flakes, prepared, whole milk & butter added	½ c	349	118
granules w/milk, prepared	½ c	246	83
granules w/out milk, prepared, whole milk & butter added	½ c	358	137
homemade w/whole milk	½ c	318	81
homemade w/whole milk & margarine	½ c	309	111
potatoes, O'Brien			
frozen, prepared	3½ oz	43	204
homemade	1 c	421	157
potatoes, scalloped			
dry mix, prepared w/whole milk & butter	5½ oz pkg	2,803	764

	Portion	Sodium (mg)	Calories
potatoes, scalloped *(cont.)*			
homemade	½ c	409	105
potato chips & sticks *See* SNACKS			
potato flour *See* FLOURS & CORNMEALS			
potato pancakes, homemade	2.7 oz	388	495
potato puffs, frozen, fried in vegetable oil	¼ oz	52	16
potato salad	½ c	661	179
sauerkraut, canned, solids & liquids	½ c	780	22
spinach soufflé	1 c	763	218

■ BRAND NAME

	Portion	Sodium (mg)	Calories
Arrowhead Mills			
potato flakes	2 oz	42	140
B&B			
mushrooms, canned	2 oz	530	25
Birds Eye Frozen Vegetables			
CHEESE SAUCE COMBINATION			
baby brussels sprouts w/cheese sauce	4½ oz	420	110
broccoli w/cheese sauce	5 oz	490	120
broccoli w/creamy Italian cheese sauce	4½ oz	390	90
cauliflower w/cheese sauce	5 oz	480	110
peas & pearl onions w/cheese sauce	5 oz	440	140
COMBINATION			
broccoli, carrots, pasta twists	3.3 oz	270	90
corn, green beans, pasta curls	3.3 oz	280	110
creamed spinach	3 oz	310	60
fresh green beans w/toasted almonds	3 oz	340	50
green peas & pearl onions	3.3 oz	440	70
green peas & potatoes w/cream sauce	2.6 oz	390	130
mixed vegetables w/onion sauce	2.6 oz	340	100
rice & green peas w/mushrooms	2.3 oz	320	110
small onions w/cream sauce	3 oz	350	110
DELUXE			
artichoke hearts	3 oz	40	30
beans, whole green	3 oz	0	25
broccoli florets	3.3 oz	20	25

	Portion	Sodium (mg)	Calories
carrots, baby peas, & pearl onions	3.3 oz	60	50
carrots, whole baby	3.3 oz	45	40
corn, tender sweet	3.3 oz	0	80
peas, tender tiny	3.3 oz	120	60

FARM FRESH MIXTURES

	Portion	Sodium (mg)	Calories
broccoli, baby carrots, water chestnuts	3.2 oz	25	35
broccoli, cauliflower, carrots	3.2 oz	25	25
broccoli, corn, red peppers	3.2 oz	15	50
broccoli, green beans, pearl onions, red peppers	3.2 oz	15	25
broccoli, red peppers, bamboo shoots, straw mushrooms	3.2 oz	15	25
brussels sprouts, cauliflower, carrots	3.2 oz	20	30
cauliflower, baby whole carrots, snow pea pods	3.2 oz	25	30

INTERNATIONAL RECIPES

	Portion	Sodium (mg)	Calories
Bavarian style	3.3 oz	420	110
Chinese style	3.3 oz	370	80
chow mein style	3.3 oz	370	90
Italian style	3.3 oz	570	110
Japanese style	3.3 oz	490	100
Mandarin style	3.3 oz	390	90
New England style	3.3 oz	410	130
pasta primavera style	3.3 oz	340	120
San Francisco style	3.3 oz	400	100

REGULAR

	Portion	Sodium (mg)	Calories
asparagus cuts	3.3 oz	5	25
beans			
baby lima	3.3 oz	115	130
cut or French cut green	3 oz	0	25
Italian green	3 oz	0	30
broccoli			
chopped	3.3 oz	15	25
cuts	3.3 oz	25	25
brussels sprouts	3.3 oz	15	35
cauliflower	3.3 oz	20	25
corn on the cob	1 ear	0	120
corn, sweet	3.3 oz	0	80
mixed vegetables	3.3 oz	40	60
onions, small whole	4 oz	10	40

	Portion	Sodium (mg)	Calories
peas, green	3.3 oz	130	80
spinach			
chopped	3.3 oz	90	20
whole leaf	3.3 oz	90	20
squash, cooked, winter	4 oz	0	45

STIR-FRY

Chinese style	3.3 oz	540	35
Japanese style	3.3 oz	510	30

Chun King

bamboo shoots	2 oz	0	16
bean sprouts	4 oz	5	40
chow mein vegetables	4 oz	20	35
water chestnuts, whole, sliced	2 oz	15	45

Claussen

sauerkraut	½ c	517	17

Fresh Chef

Holiday cole slaw	4 oz	214	199
Old Fashioned potato salad	4 oz	320	210

Joan of Arc

garden salad	½ c	500	70
potato salad			
German style	½ c	550	120
Home Style	½ c	535	170
yams			
in orange pineapple sauce	½ c	15	190
mashed	½ c	45	90
whole, packed in heavy syrup	½ c	15	120

Le Sueur
FROZEN, IN BUTTER SAUCE

early peas	½ c	520	70
minipeas, pea pods, & water chestnuts	½ c	410	80
peas, carrots, & onions	½ c	470	80

Mexicorn

Mexicorn w/peppers	½ c	310	80

Mrs. Paul's Prepared Vegetables

candied sweet potatoes	4 oz	60	190
corn fritters	2	630	250
eggplant parmigiana	5 oz	600	260
fried eggplant sticks	3½ oz	610	240
onion rings, crispy	2½ oz	270	180
zucchini sticks, light batter	3 oz	440	200

	Portion	Sodium (mg)	Calories
Ortega			
green chiles, whole, diced, strips, sliced	1 oz	20	10
hot peppers, whole, diced	1 oz	0	8
jalapeño peppers, whole, diced	1 oz	20	10
tomatoes & jalapeños	1 oz	120	8
Pillsbury			
BUTTER SAUCE VEGETABLES			
baby lima beans	½ c	460	110
broccoli spears	½ c	340	45
brussels sprouts	½ c	260	40
cut green beans	½ c	210	30
cut leaf spinach	½ c	470	45
French-style green beans	½ c	360	35
mixed vegetables	½ c	330	70
Niblets corn	½ c	280	100
sweet peas	½ c	430	80
CANNED VEGETABLES			
asparagus cuts/spears	½ c	420	20
cream-style corn	½ c	390	100
cut green beans	½ c	300	20
mushrooms	½ c	430	25
mushrooms in butter sauce	2 oz	330	30
sweet peas	½ c	320	50
sweet peas & onions	½ c	510	50
three-bean salad	½ c	410	70
whole kernel corn, vacuum pack	½ c	28	80
CREAM & CHEESE SAUCE COMBINATION			
baby brussels sprouts in cheese-flavored sauce	½ c	510	70
broccoli cauliflower carrots in cheese-flavored sauce	½ c	490	70
broccoli in cheese-flavored sauce	½ c	530	60
broccoli in white cheddar cheese–flavored sauce	½ c	450	50
cauliflower in cheese-flavored sauce	½ c	500	60
cauliflower in white cheddar cheese–flavored sauce	½ c	390	50
cream-style corn	½ c	370	110
creamed spinach	½ c	480	80
peas in cream sauce	½ c	320	90
HARVEST FRESH			
broccoli spears	½ c	190	20
cut broccoli	½ c	150	18

	Portion	Sodium (mg)	Calories
cut green beans	½ c	150	16
early June peas	½ c	170	60
lima beans	½ c	210	60
mixed vegetables	½ c	160	45
Niblets corn	½ c	140	80
spinach	½ c	340	25
sweet peas	½ c	200	50
POLYBAG VEGETABLES			
broccoli cuts	½ c	15	12
brussels sprouts	½ c	10	25
cauliflower cuts	½ c	25	12
green beans	½ c	10	14
lima beans	½ c	30	100
mixed vegetables	½ c	30	50
Niblets corn	½ c	5	80
Niblets corn on the cob	1 ear	20	150
sweet peas	½ c	15	50
POTATO SIDE DISHES			
stuffed baked potato w/cheese-flavored topping	1	520	200
stuffed baked potato w/sour cream & chives	1	580	230
VALLEY COMBINATION DUAL POUCH W/SAUCE			
American-style vegetables	½ c	240	70
Broccoli Cauliflower Medley	½ c	260	50
Broccoli Fanfare	½ c	330	70
Italian-style vegetables	½ c	220	40
Japanese-style vegetables	½ c	420	45
Le Sueur–style vegetables	½ c	330	60
Mexican-style vegetables	½ c	400	140
VALLEY COMBINATIONS, POLYBAG			
Broccoli Carrot Fanfare	½ c	30	20
Broccoli Cauliflower Supreme	½ c	30	20
Cauliflower Green Bean Festival	½ c	30	16
Corn Broccoli Bounty	½ c	15	45
Sweet Pea Cauliflower Medley	½ c	60	30
Vlasic			
Old Fashioned sauerkraut	1 oz	280	4

□ **VINEGAR** *See* **SALAD DRESSINGS, MAYONNAISE, VINEGAR, & DIPS**

	Portion	Sodium (mg)	Calories

□ **WHEY** *See* MILK, MILK SUBSTITUTES, & MILK PRODUCTS

□ **YOGURT** *See* MILK, MILK SUBSTITUTES, & MILK PRODUCTS

□ **YOGURT, FROZEN** *See* DESSERTS, FROZEN